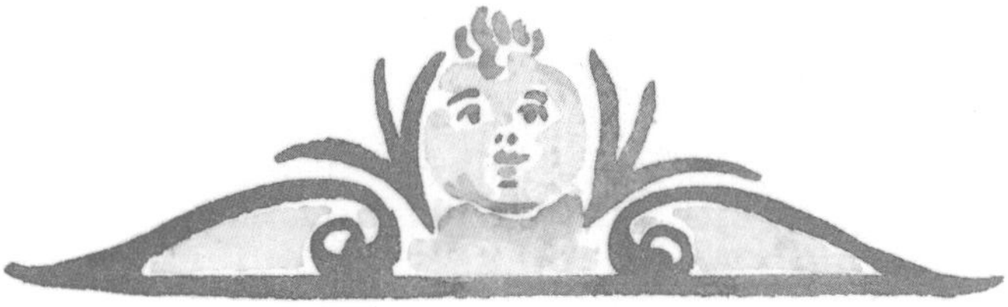

· LETTERS ·
TO A CHILD
BEING BORN

A pregnancy journal with quotes, sentiments, and space for writing

Written and compiled by Karen Scott Boates

RUNNING PRESS
Philadelphia, Pennsylvania

Canadian representatives: General Publishing Co., Ltd., 30 Lesmill Road, Don Mills, Ontario M3B 2T6. International representatives: Worldwide Media Services, Inc., 115 East Twenty-third Street, New York, New York 10010.

ISBN 1-56138-046-6
Cover design by Toby Schmidt
Cover illustration by Kimmerle Milnazik
Interior design by Nancy Loggins
Interior illustrations by Lisa Umlauf-Roese
Typography: ITC Garamond Light and Antique Olive by
Commcor Communications Corporation, Philadelphia, Pennsylvania

Excerpt from "Spring Tide" by Summer Brenner, published in a collection of poems, *From the Heart to the Center*, The Figures, 1977, reprinted by permission of Summer Brenner. Excerpt from "Birth" reprinted by permission of Madeline Tiger; complete poem appears in the following collections: *Toward Spring Bank*, © 1981 by Madeline Tiger, Damascus Road Press, and the anthology *The Limits of MIRACLES, Poems about the Loss of Babies*, collected by Marion Deutsche Cohen, Bergin & Garvey Publishers, Inc., Massachusetts, 1985. Sharon Olds: "The Planned Child" © 1985 by Sharon Olds, originally published in *Poetry* magazine, reprinted by permission of the author. Excerpt from "Natural Birth" reprinted by permission of Toi Derricotte; complete poem appears in *Natural Birth*, © 1983 by Toi Derricotte, Crossing Press. Excerpt from "The Language of the Brag" reprinted from *Satan Says*, by Sharon Olds, by permission of the University of Pittsburgh Press, © 1980 by Sharon Olds.

This book may be ordered by mail from the publisher.
Please add $2.50 for postage and handling.
But try your bookstore first!
Running Press Book Publishers
125 South Twenty-second Street
Philadelphia, Pennsylvania 19103

Introduction

For the Womb has dreams.

It is not as simple as the good earth.

ANAÏS NIN (1903–1977)
The Diary of Anaïs Nin

We are consumed by the thought, and then the knowledge of pregnancy. After we plan, think, wonder, and try—at some point during the first few days, weeks, or months—most of us become aware of this private internal drama. As our body embraces the child to be, the very idea of creating new life encircles us, sweeps us up, and changes us forever.

Anaïs Nin said, "For the Womb has dreams," and indeed, that dark sleeping center, now touched by the spark of creation, becomes a whooshing, whomping factory of life, and we dream about possibility and potential. Women tend to fall in love with this potential almost from the moment of conception, and the love, hopes, and fears expressed in our dreams reveal to us the collective stories of all women. Stories telling of continuity of generations, changes brought to our own lives, and glimpses of the one fragile human life entrusted to us.

What a job for just one person! We watch other pregnant women so carefully, hoping to see mirrored in them this force that has us in its gentle grips—slowly, slowly gaining power. And then we have the realization that there is only one way out—My God!

Pregnancy lasts just forty weeks, a period when a mother, as well as a child, is emerging. Many experiences at this time are common to all women: confirmation of the pregnancy, physical transformation, preparation for birth. But many other experiences are entirely personal, a gestalt of the individual history you bring to this unique experience. Unique because this time it is happening to you alone.

So it is with the journal you are holding. The quotes and letters in this journal articulate the commonality of pregnancy and birth, the sisterhood of collective sentiment. The blank pages offer you a place to record your individual feelings, poems, drawings, and dreams.

As the author of this journal you will create a gift. The gift is to yourself and to the child you carry, for the two of you are intertwined, and the distinction at this point between mother and child is a false one. Speak to your child, whisper those dreams, fears, and hopes as they come to you, and pen a diary of this exceptional time in both of your lives.

KAREN SCOTT BOATES

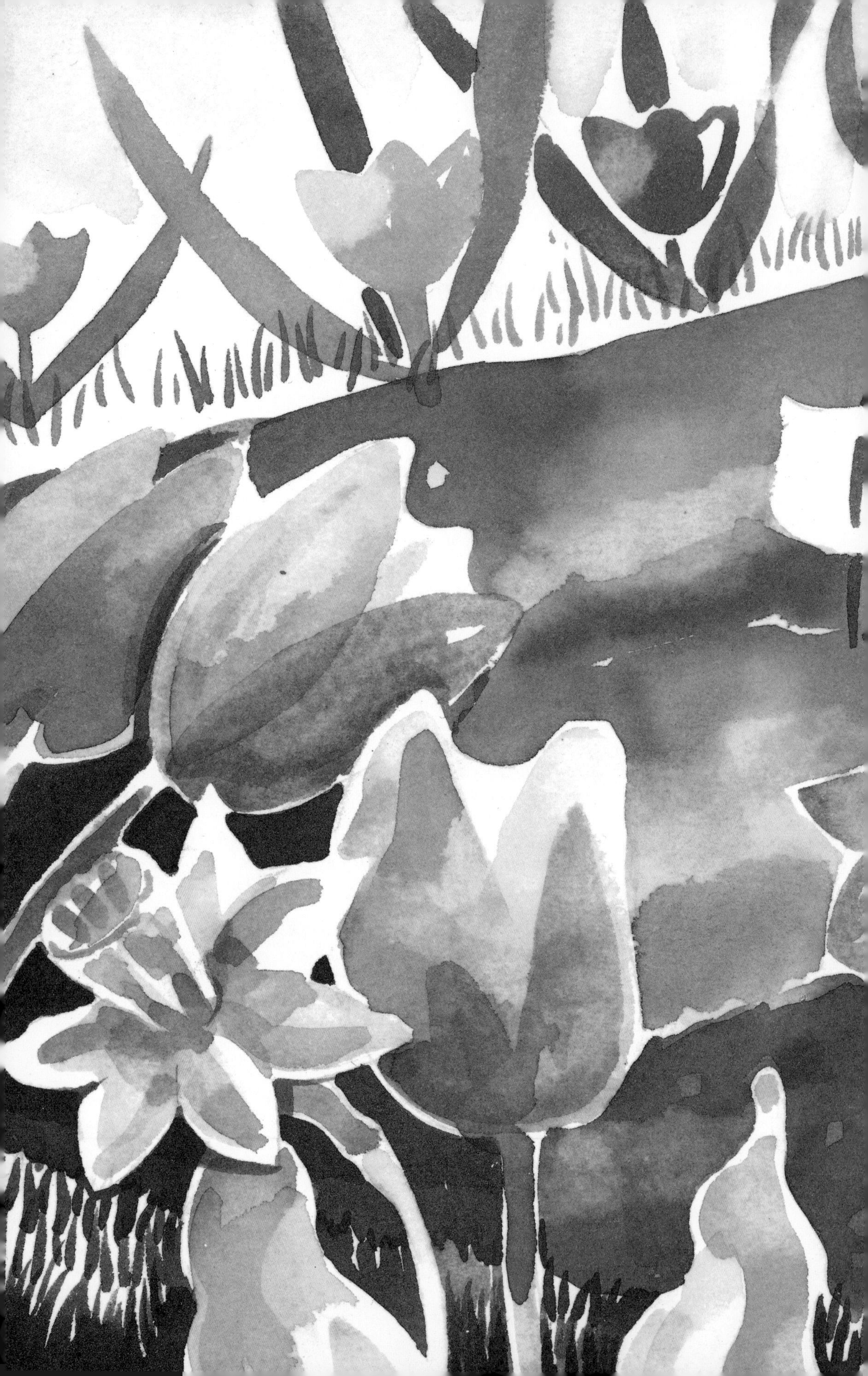

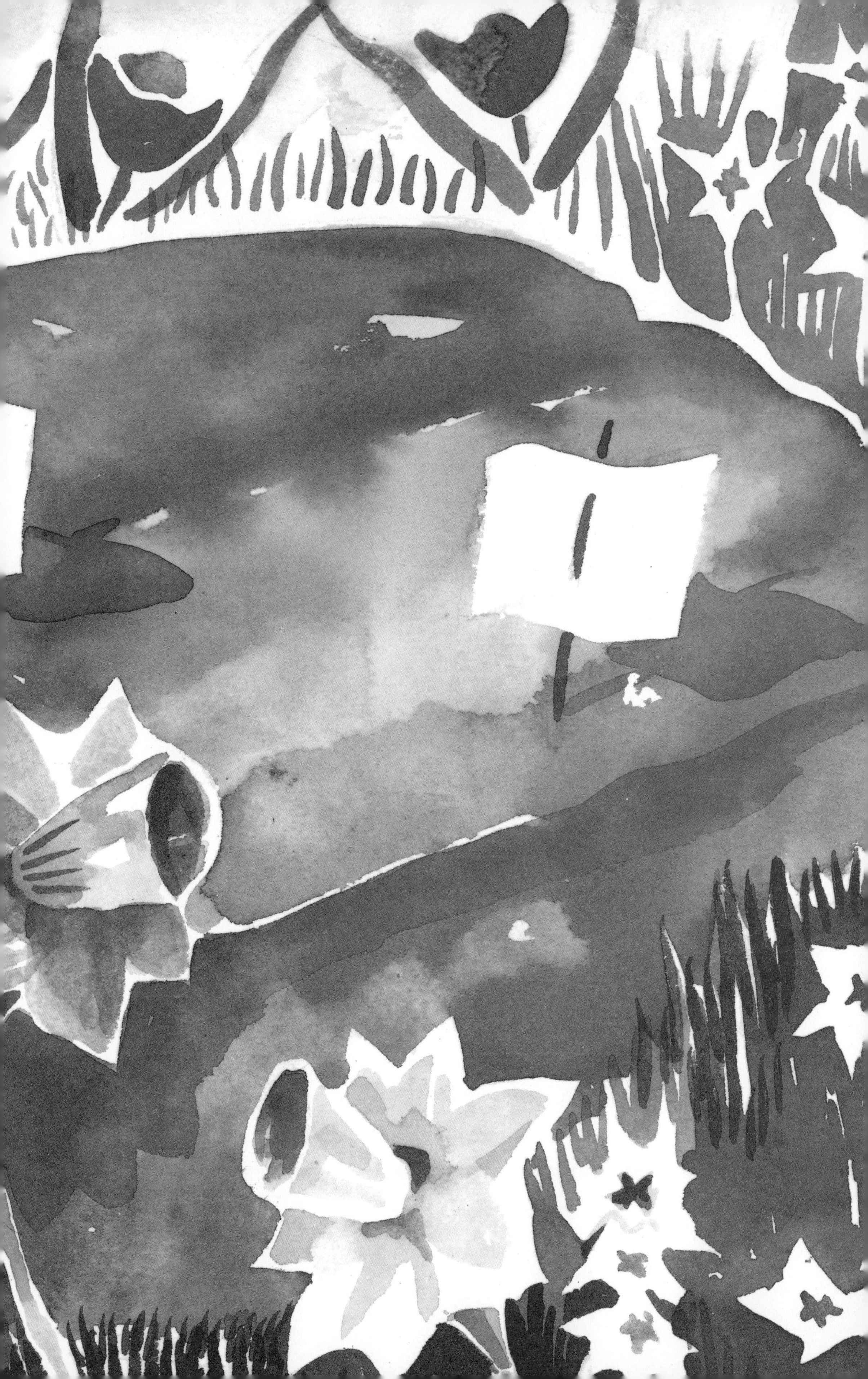

1

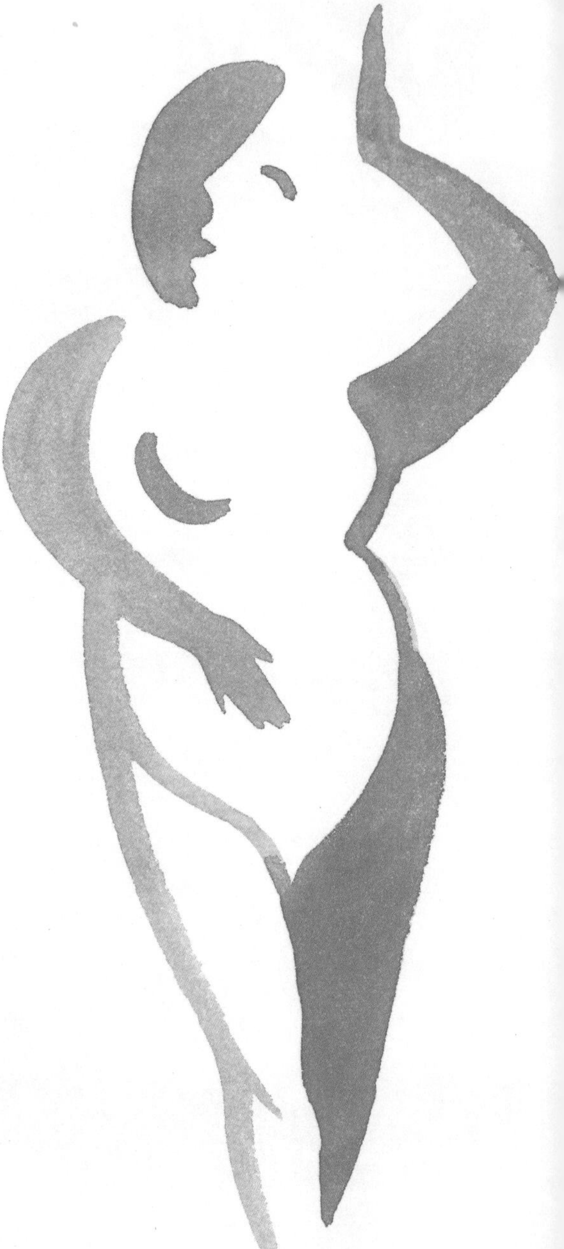

If a little feeling of pain
doth runne up and downe the lower
belly and about the navell, if shee
be sleepy, if she loath the embracing
of a man, and if her face bee pale, it
is a token that she hath conceived.

AMBROISE PARÉ
Collected Works

Upon Confirmation

It's true. Expecting company and so much more!

You exist. Where did you come from? Did a part of me know already, when I heard the explosion and felt the rumblings, deep within, echoes of creation? Was that you, making such a racket, seedling of two souls joined together?

It's not every morning that one wakes to find oneself in the middle of a miracle. It is said dry crackers first thing in the morning make a miracle more comfortable.

1

1

1

2

There is man-made importance
and there is the lunar egg.

And in that scarlet orb
almost feathered for conception
there are no illusions of immortality
Only a whiney yolk
to perhaps improbably
further on the species
So precisely every 28 days
we women house a miscellaneous creation
that there in the painful cotton
we are reminded of tides
corn growing in season
ageless labors and ancient orders
fixing us in the tradition of an acorn
We pass life
and it is garbage
it is graceful waste
it is falling off the roof
as my mother calls it
An opening that bleeds
passing rhythm of seasons
musical blood

There is no pretense on the pad
It is biological failure
The ovary is dutiful not ambitious
It just accidentally fructates the mensual connection
of love for what is life and death

O Isis
my Mississippi
my delta

SUMMER BRENNER
"Spring Tide"

Each month the nest is prepared and then with the biological discovery that no one is home, house cleaning commences.

This month that rhythm halts. Well, come, tiny sprout, make yourself a home.

2

2

2

2

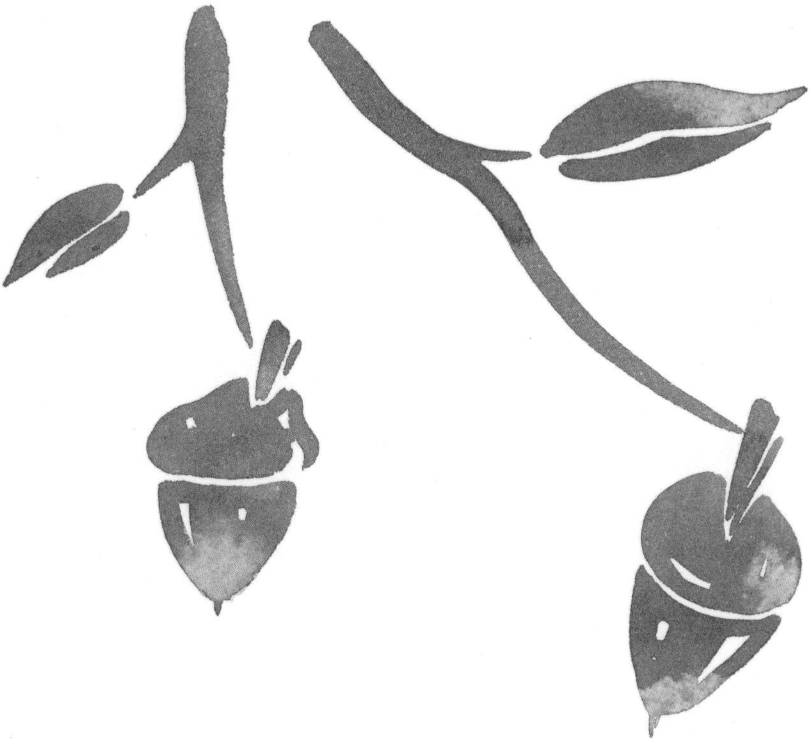

Mothers of daughters are daughters of mothers and have remained so, in circles joined to circles, since time began. They are bound together by a shared destiny. Daughters have been expected simply to assume the identity of their mothers, "naturally" growing up to become wives and mothers in their "own right." The sense of biological inevitability underlying this expectation has been taken for granted by both sexes until quite recently; in fact, the generation of daughters now growing up may be the first one in history to feel that motherhood can be one choice among many that a woman can make.

SIGNE HAMMER
Mothers and Daughters

3

Choice

Today we have choice, even if our choice is not to choose. I decide for the rest of my life and yours.

A friend reminded me that every acorn which falls from the tree does not grow to be an oak. Well, I choose to grow the oak, to keep this acorn planted, and the gentle winds and later storms will teach us together.

Remember, even little babies make choices. Have you chosen your nose yet?

3

3

3

Telling

So we made Nancy promise not to tell anyone, especially not Kate. We didn't want our friend to mistrust us. So now Nancy knows, and Kate doesn't know, plus Kate's mother knows and Mel doesn't know, and neither does Kate's father.

But what if Nancy accidentally told Mel that Kate had told her mother, having to explain that it was just something a daughter couldn't keep back, but that he shouldn't let on that he knew that Kate's mother knew, so that Kate would finally be the only one who didn't know what.

LAURA CHESTER
"Who Knows" in *Cradle and All*

4

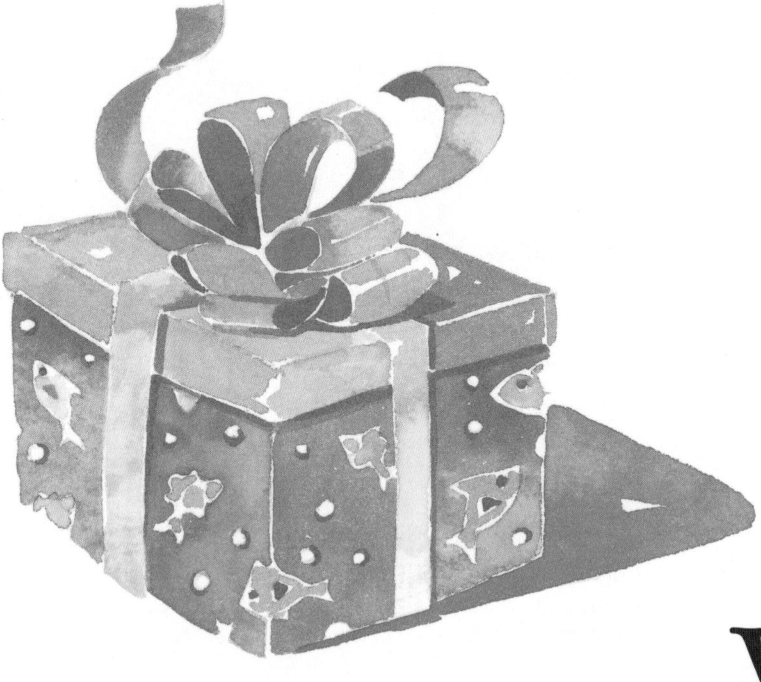

Who shall we tell, Little One? Perhaps just the two of us will keep this secret for a little while longer. No, I think that's impossible. How can they look at us and not see the shout of your being? Can't they hear a revolution is going on?

4

4

4

4

Due Date

The average pregnancy is 266 days long. . . .

MIRIAM STOPPARD, M.D.
Dr. Miriam Stoppard's Pregnancy and Birth Book

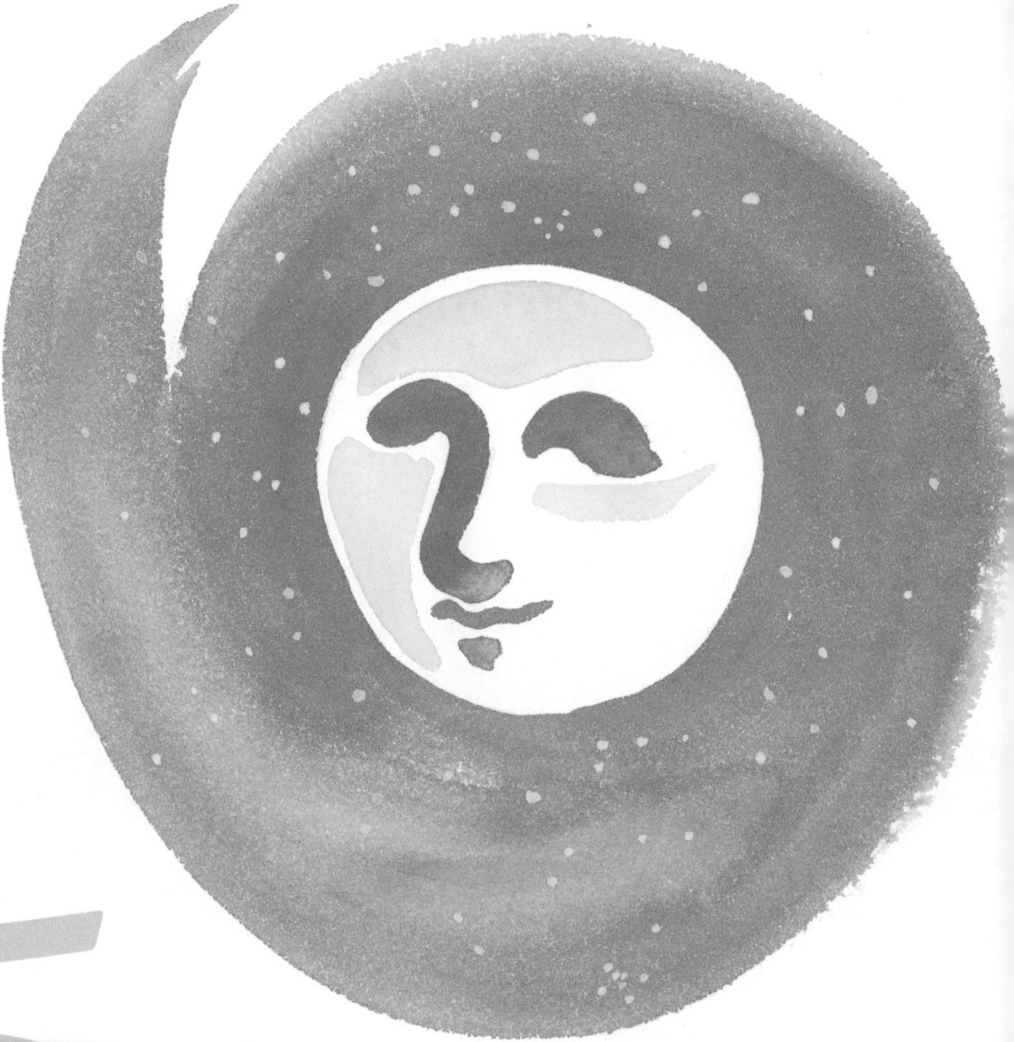

5

Due Date

5

First day of the last menstrual cle, plus nine months, plus seven days. And when that day arrives, will u? No mother has an "average" pregnancy, and babies don't come with calendar. The time of arrival is counted by the moon and inner tides.

The day of your birth does not belong to us personally. At that oment, we are an instrument played by Life itself.

5

5

6

The Heart

What is the human body but a constellation of the same powers that formed the stars in the sky?

PARACLESUS

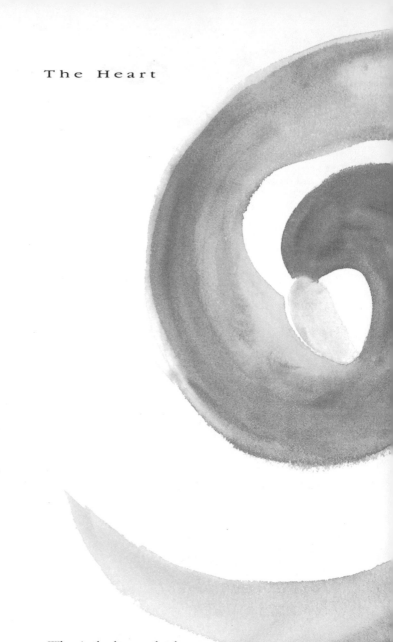

The Heart

6

At six weeks your arms re so short they cannot even fold over the red speck in the center of your hest. That spot, your heart, beats one hundred and fifty times a minute, wice as fast as mine.

In my mind's eye I see our hearts as an interlocking valentine, eating a syncopated rhythm of growth and vitality.

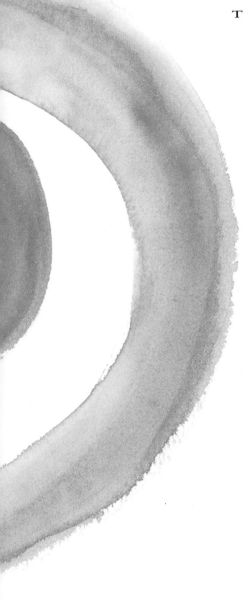

6

6

6

Origins

7

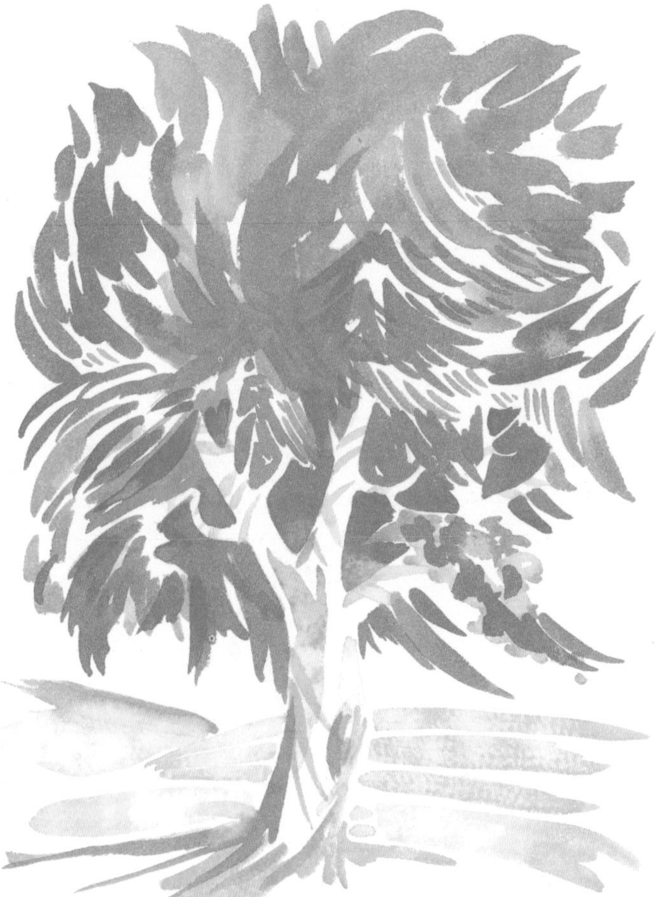

Our birth is but a sleep and a forgetting:
The Soul that rises with us, our life's Star,
Hath had elsewhere its setting,
And cometh from afar.

WILLIAM WORDSWORTH
"Ode, Intimations of Immortality"

7

According to Plato, you soul lived somewhere else before you joined me, and all knowledge brought from that other life in the form of recollection. He said that babie know the most because they haven't had as much time to forget.

According to Plato, you are wiser than I. Good thing.

7

7

Mechanics

8

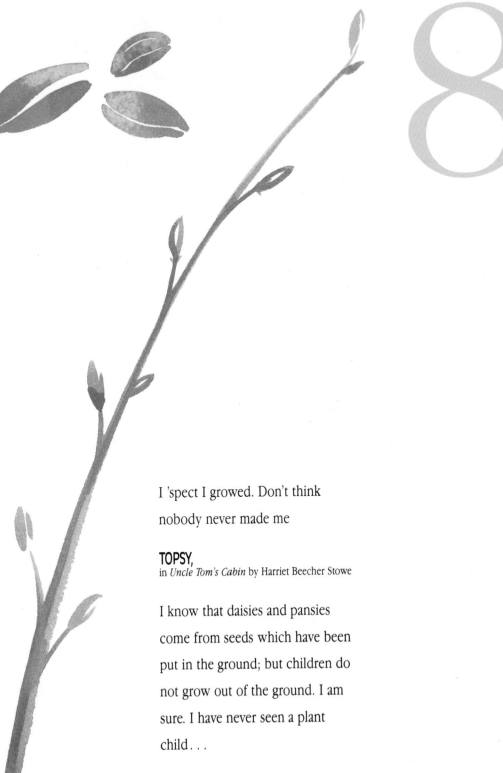

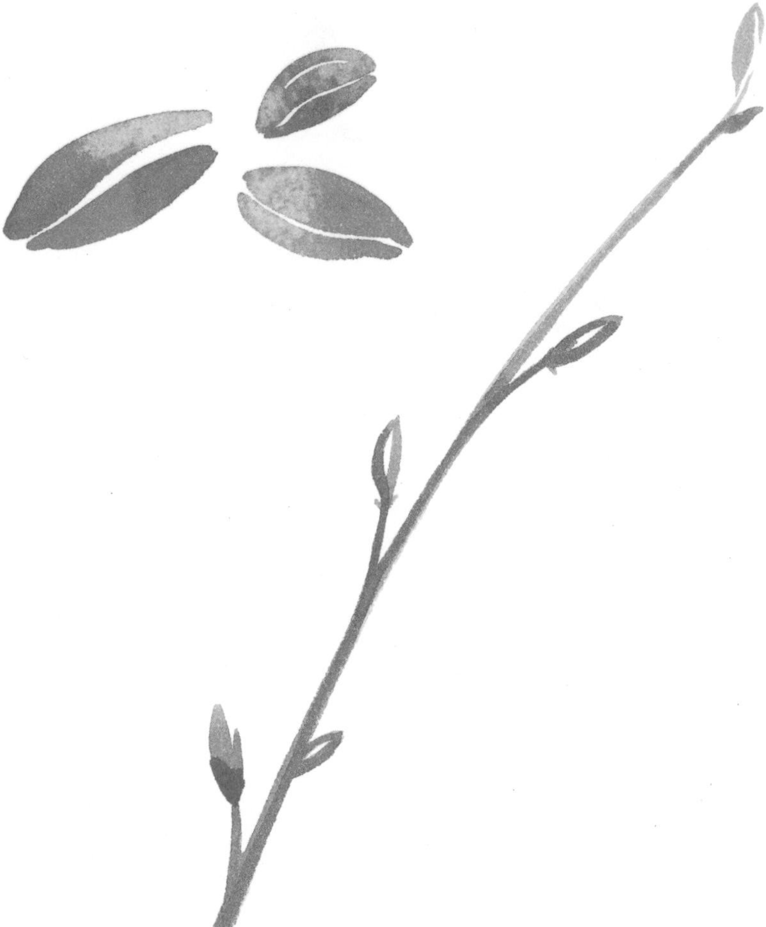

I 'spect I growed. Don't think nobody never made me

TOPSY,
in *Uncle Tom's Cabin* by Harriet Beecher Stowe

I know that daisies and pansies come from seeds which have been put in the ground; but children do not grow out of the ground. I am sure. I have never seen a plant child . . .

HELEN KELLER
The Story of My Life

8

Mechanics

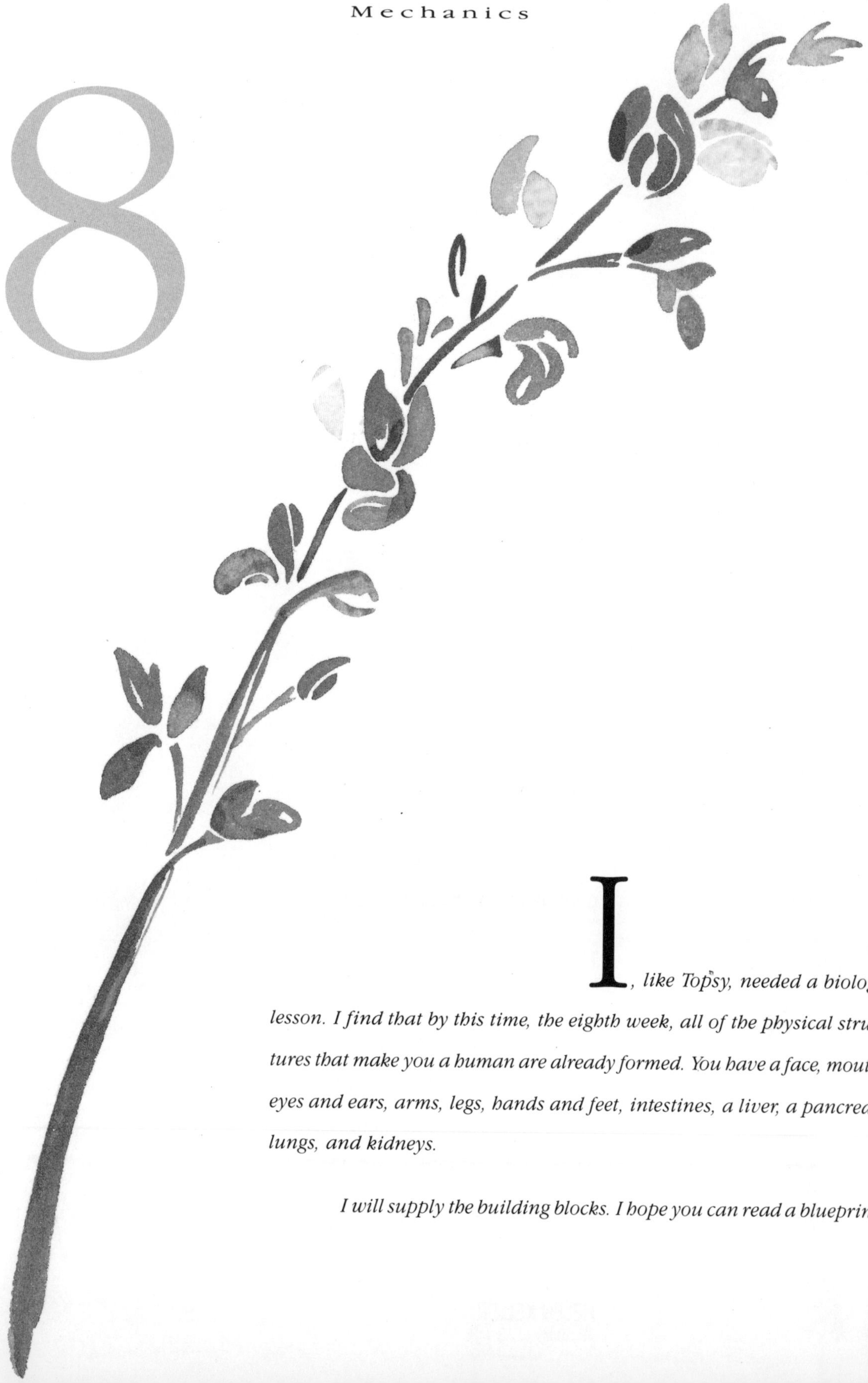

I, like Topsy, needed a biology lesson. I find that by this time, the eighth week, all of the physical structures that make you a human are already formed. You have a face, mouth, eyes and ears, arms, legs, hands and feet, intestines, a liver, a pancreas, lungs, and kidneys.

I will supply the building blocks. I hope you can read a blueprint.

8

8

9

Once upon a time a beautiful young lady and a very handsome young man fell in love and got married. They were a wonderful, compatible couple, and God blessed the marriage with a fine baby boy (eight pounds eight ounces). They loved their little boy very much. They raised him, nurtured him, and spoiled him. They raised him in the palm of the hand and gave him everything they thought he wanted. Finally, when he was about seven or eight, they let his feet touch the ground.

DUKE ELLINGTON
Music is My Mistress

It's a girl . . .a little beauty,
an angel, and I'm madly in love
with her.

HENRY MILLER,
on the birth of his daughter

A Boy or Girl

9

People ask, "Do you want a boy or a girl?"

The answer is "Yes, of course."

9

9

10

To be "born of a white hen" was to be "born with a silver spoon in the mouth," "child of fortune," or "fortune's favorite." Suetonius gives the origin of the proverb. When Livia, wife of Augustus Caesar, was at one of her country seats, an eagle flying over the place dropped a white hen, holding a sprig of laurel in its beak, into her lap. The Empress was so pleased with the adventure that she ordered the hen to be well taken care of and the laurel to be planted in the garden. Both prospered, and branches from the laurel were used for many years by the emperors in their triumphs.

JUVENAL
Satires

10

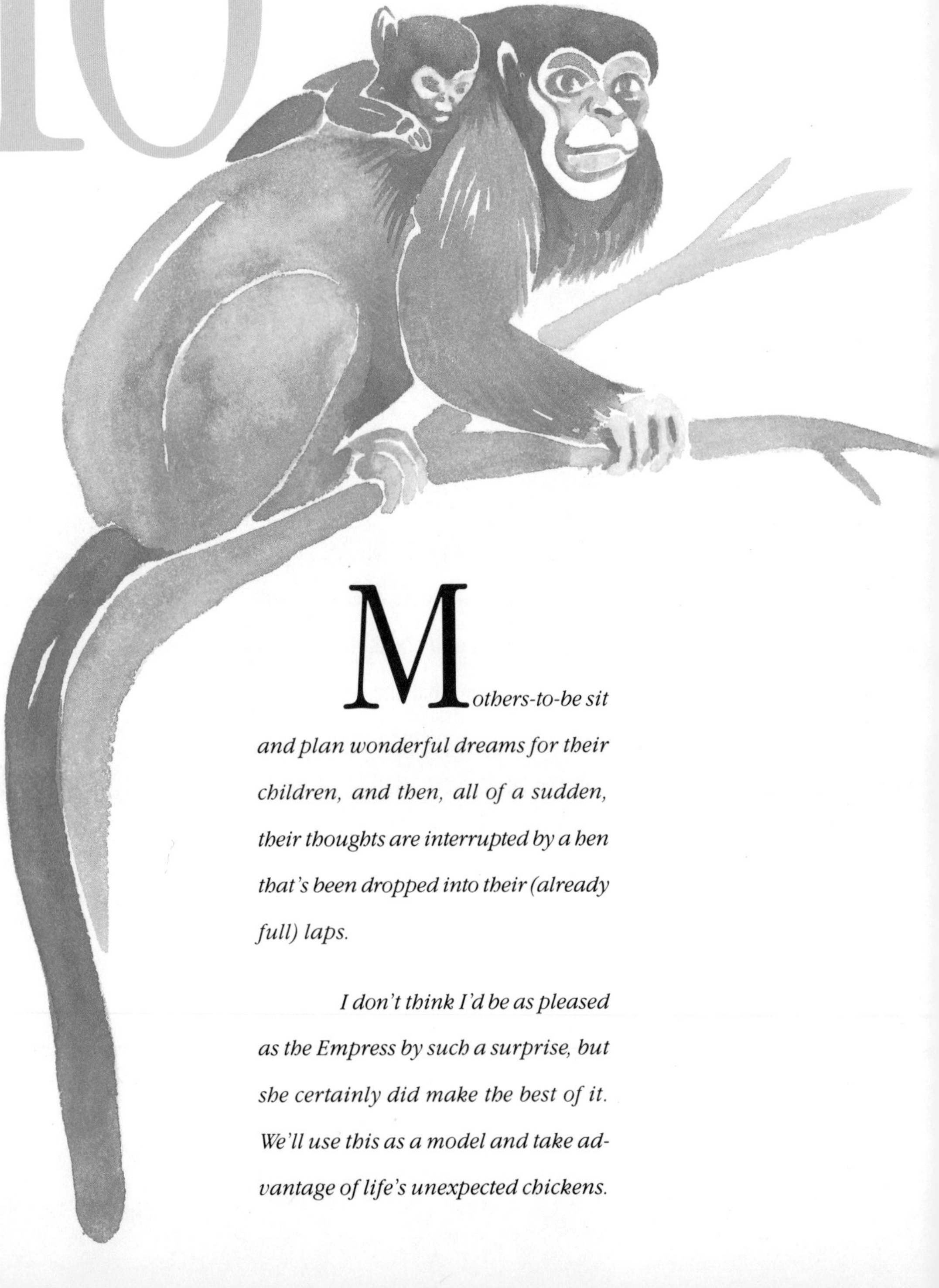

Mothers-to-be sit and plan wonderful dreams for their children, and then, all of a sudden, their thoughts are interrupted by a hen that's been dropped into their (already full) laps.

I don't think I'd be as pleased as the Empress by such a surprise, but she certainly did make the best of it. We'll use this as a model and take advantage of life's unexpected chickens.

10

10

10

Names

11

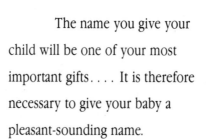

The name you give your child will be one of your most important gifts. . . . It is therefore necessary to give your baby a pleasant-sounding name.

LAREINA RULE
Name Your Baby

There are 50,000 Mary Smiths and an equal number of John Smiths in this country, according to the Social Security Administration. There is one John 5/8 Smith.

Harry S Truman's S is just an S.

BRUCE LANSKY
10,000 Baby Names

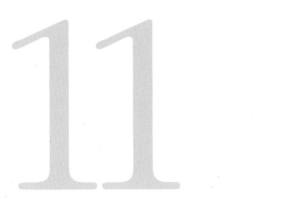

11

I *love baby name books—the oys' names and the girls' names, the names for both and some definitely or neither. Such personality and potential. I hold a gift from our ances-ors—the power of naming, of placing the history of past generations upon our shoulders so you will know who you are and where you've come from.*

Or perhaps I shall give you a fresh start and we'll snatch from this noment just the right sound. We could make one up. Send me some letters n a dream. I'll string them like beads into the perfect name and mono-ram the sky for you.

11

11

12

Storks are proverbially devoted to their young. When a thatched roof caught fire in Denmark a few years ago, the mother bird stuck to her nest, covering her young and, as the flames rolled nearer, beating her wings violently to keep the youngsters from suffocating in the smoke. When the fire was extinguished, she was black with soot, but her babies were saved.

Small wonder that the baby-bringing legend attached itself to this tender fowl. And that belief is not so silly as it sounds. For the original thought was that the stork who came to preside on the family roof embodied the soul of some ancestor and took the liveliest interest in each anticipated descendant. So he it was, people came to think, who fetched, from that well or spring the village called "the children's fountain," not the expected baby's body but its little soul.

DONALD CULROSS PEATTIE
"The Story of the Stork"

The Stork

With or without the stork, it seems to me pregnancy and birth is a journey from the mystery of night to the greater mystery of day.

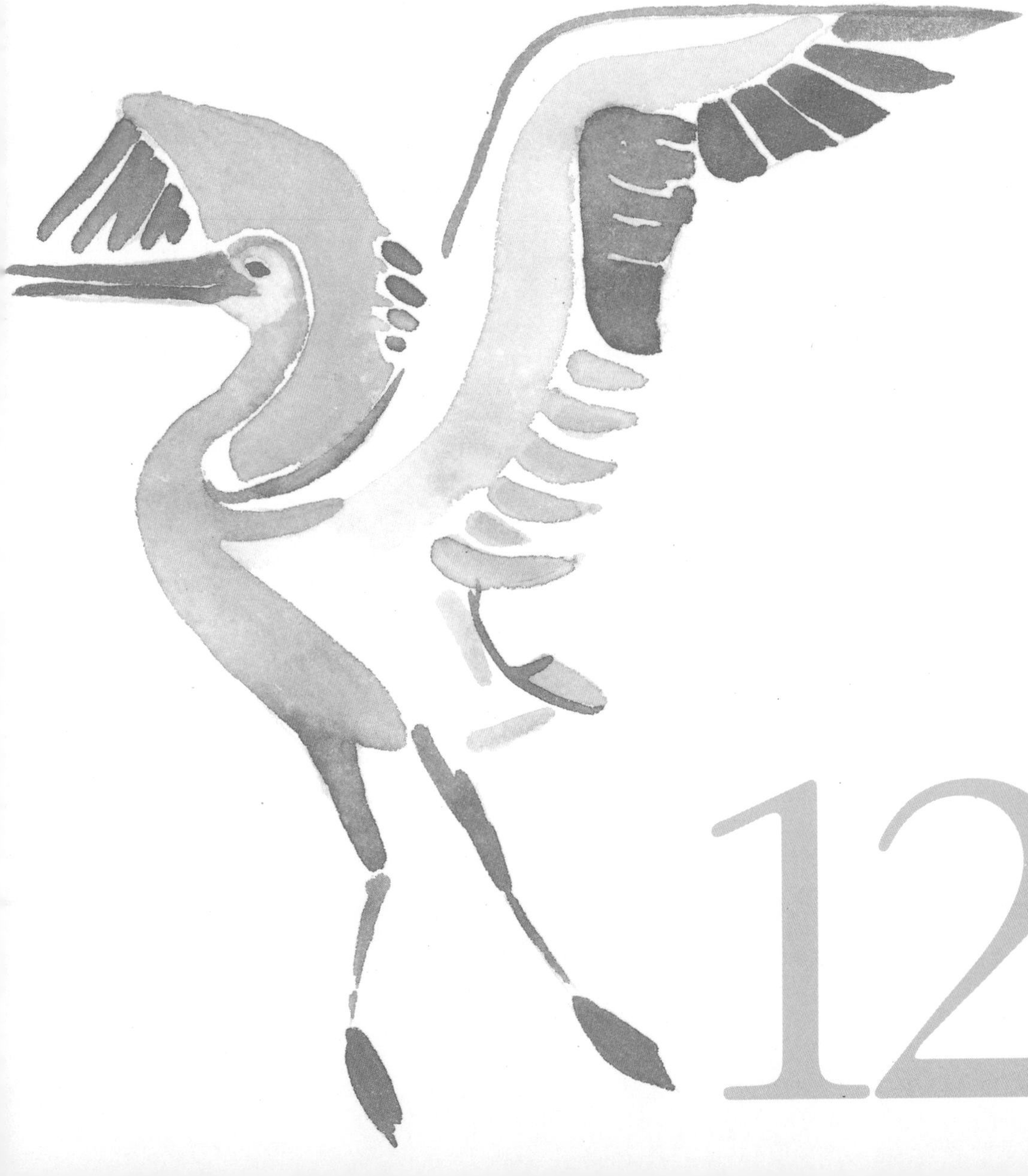

12

12

12

12

The Mossi of the Sudan prayed [to their ancestors] for large families at earth shrines where there are landmarks such as trees, mountains, rocks, or rivers. The priests of the shrines intercede for the people, and if this is correctly done the spiritual agents of the ancestors pass into the wombs of women and are born as children.

ELLIOT P. SKINNER
Gods and Rituals

Generations

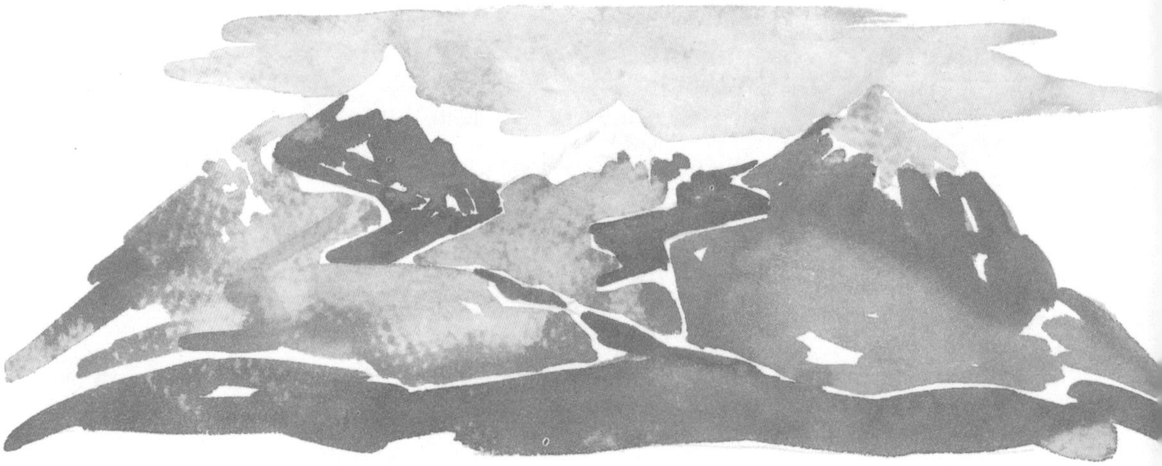

Is this why so many babies loo like wizened old men? Will it really be the countenance of a grea grandfather traced over my new child's face?

Through the similarity of features and traits, you and I hol hands across time. The impact of your birth, so significant to our famil links us in a double helix of generations.

13

13

13

13

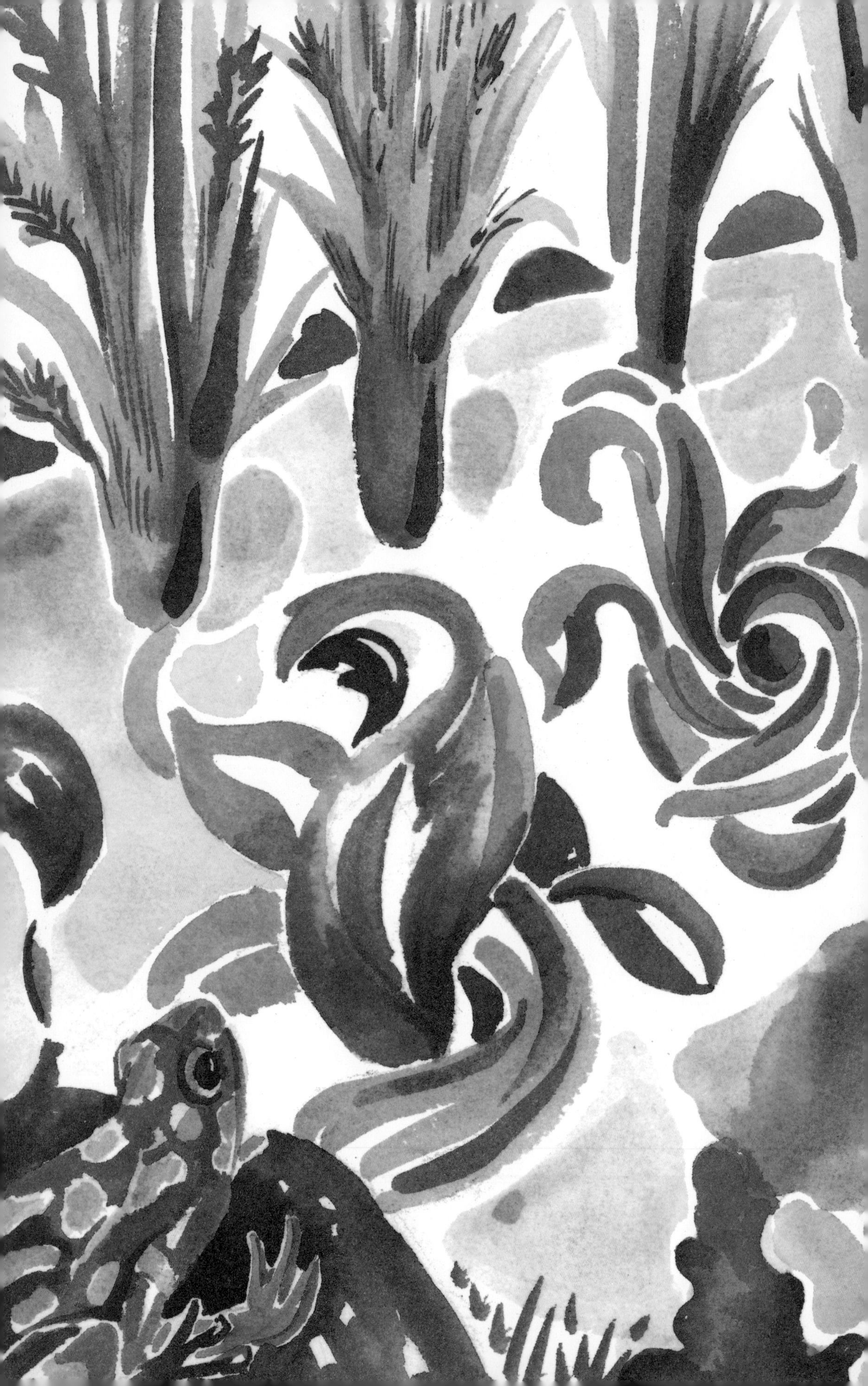

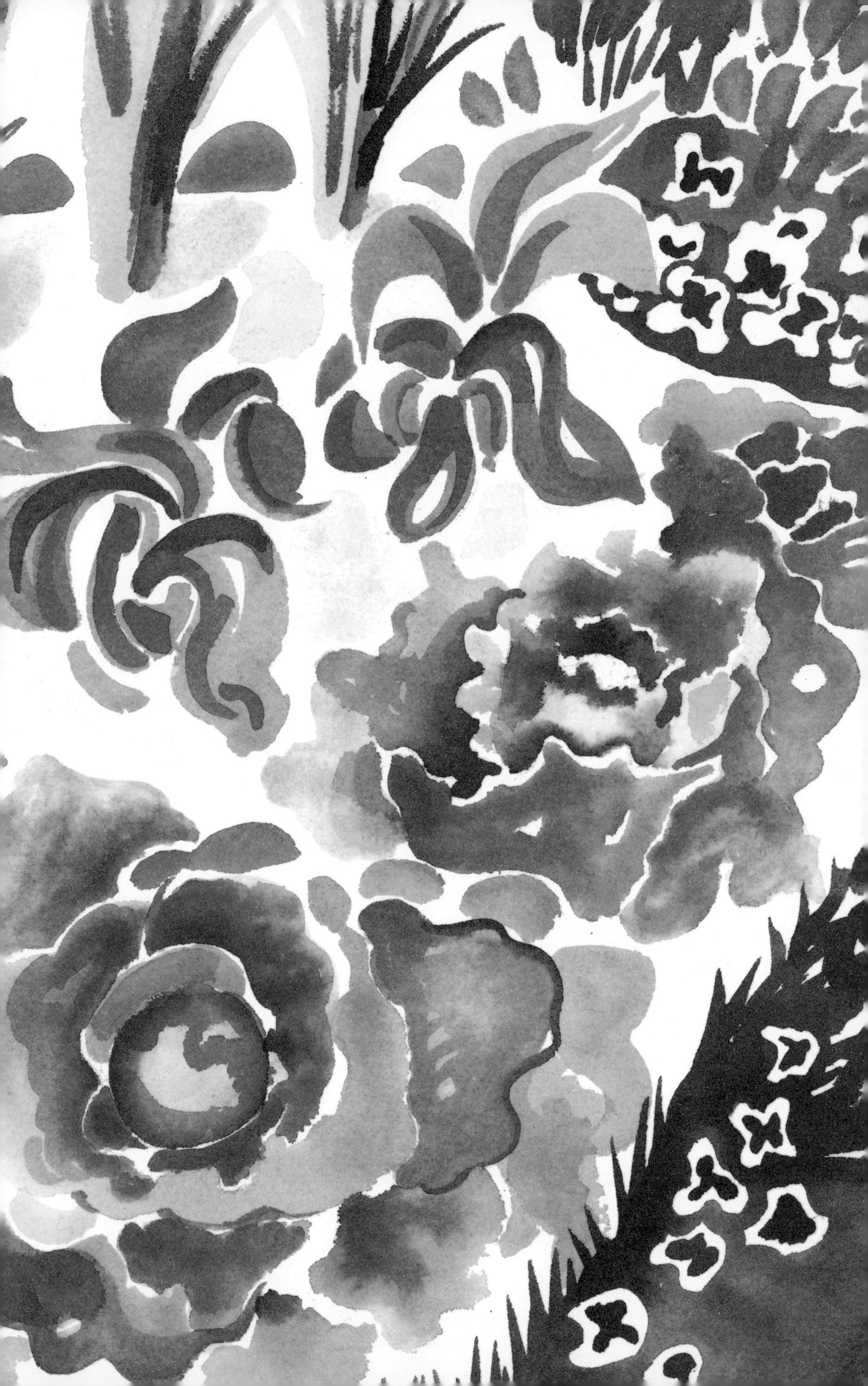

Although you don't have to agree to carry it for her, you *should* make an effort to keep helping her and to keep expressing your love. Make sure that she sits in comfortable chairs; and then help her out of the chair when it's time to leave, or else you'll find yourself in the street without her because she'll still be in the chair, flapping her arms and trying to get airborne.

BILL COSBY
Fatherhood

14

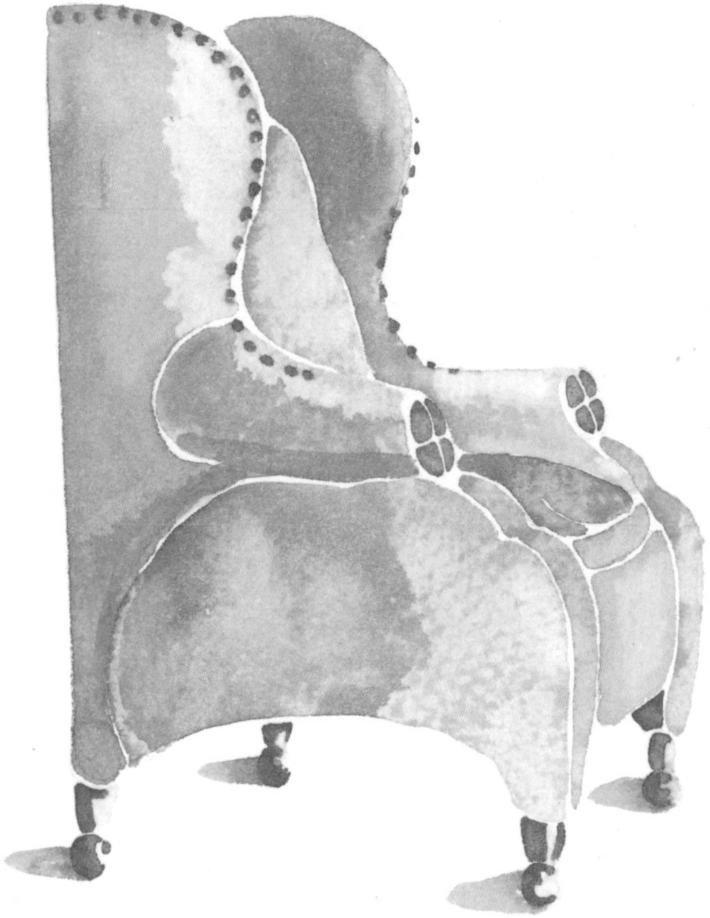

Do I still look beautiful to your father, or ugly, or just silly? Physically I'm pregnant, but psychologically we both are. Is his mind expanding as much as my belly?

Let's all go shopping together and I'll buy him a maternity hat.

14

14

14

Couvade

15

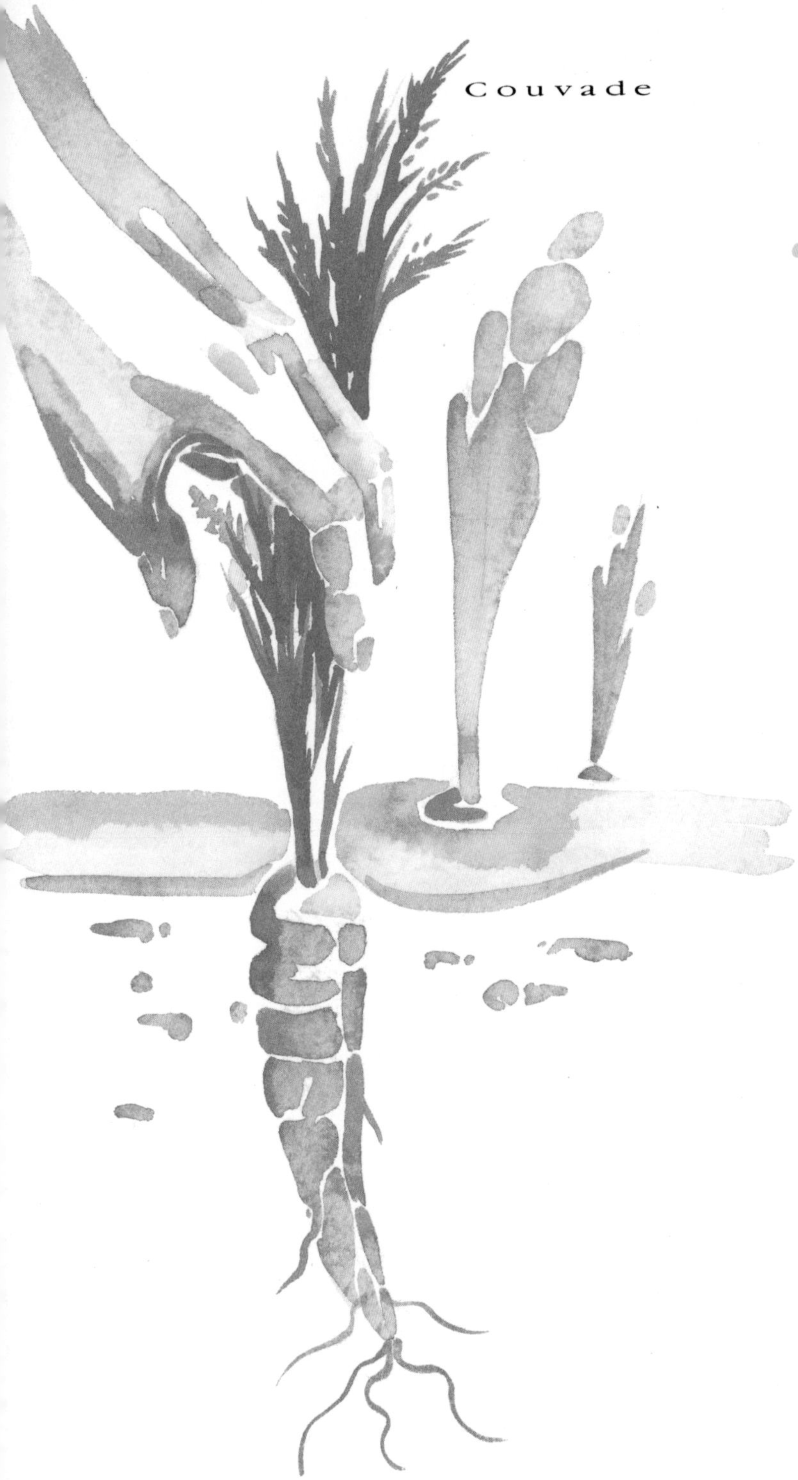

During the first trimester of my wife's pregnancy with our son, her weight stayed the same and I put on 10 pounds.

LAWRENCE KUTNER
The New York Times

Couvade

15

Couvade *is a French ter*
which means "to hatch." It is the name given to a custom prevalent amon
some primitive tribes in which the father goes to bed and experiences labo
while his wife is bearing the child.

Today, various studies claim anywhere from 11% to 65% of ex
pectant fathers experience the couvade syndrome during their wives' preg
nancies. Especially in the third month, and again during the birth of th
child, the father may experience any or all of the symptoms associated wit
a normal pregnancy. This appears to be a positive sign that a family
truly emerging.

15

15

16

I ran into a woman from town whom I know only by sight. She stopped me to remark about how fit and pink I was looking and asked how things were going. She told me about her own good times during the last couple of months of pregnancy. I told her about my boundless energy, now that things are really underway, and my desire to clean and cook and sew. She nodded and smiled. . . . We stood on the street, not knowing each other's name, and felt very close.

SUZANNE ARMS
A Season to be Born

16

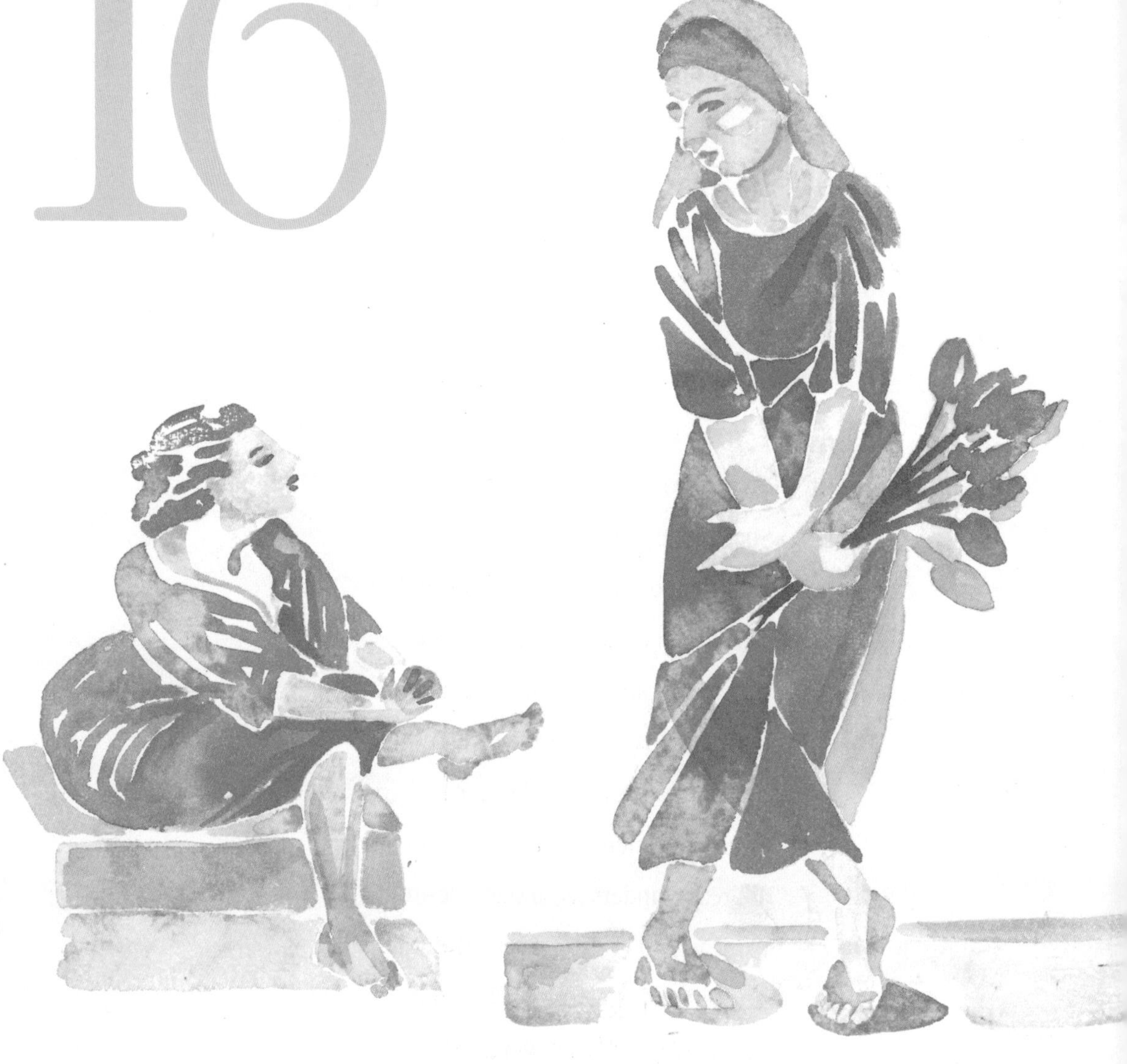

Old wives seem so wise to me now. I search each of their tales for the bits of truth they hold.

I don't even know the questions to ask about mothering except this one—after you are here, who will mother me?

16

16

16

17

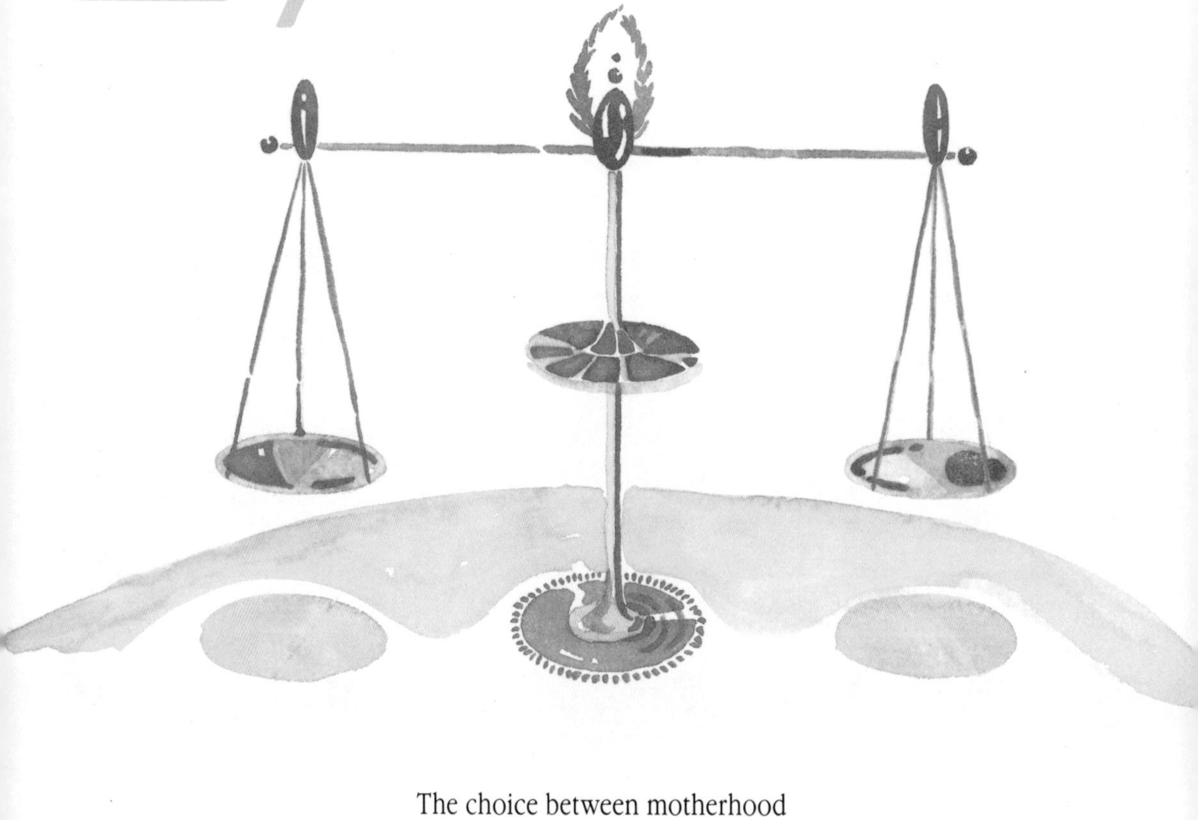

The choice between motherhood and selfhood is a false one; it need not be made. Neither mother nor child can thrive at the expense of the other.

LYN DELLIQUADRI AND KATI BRECKENRIDGE
Mothercare

All mothers are working mothers.

But still there are decisions to be made about your care, my care, career, and money. The scales have been upset and must be realigned. As I study the balance of hours and years, I realize we have a lifetime to include everything I want for the two of us.

17

17

18

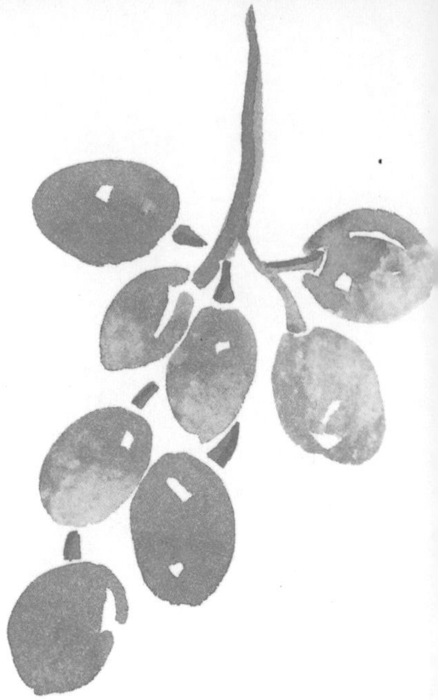

We all used to care so much about what we didn't eat; these days, it's so much more sane—we care about what we do eat.

DONNA KARAN

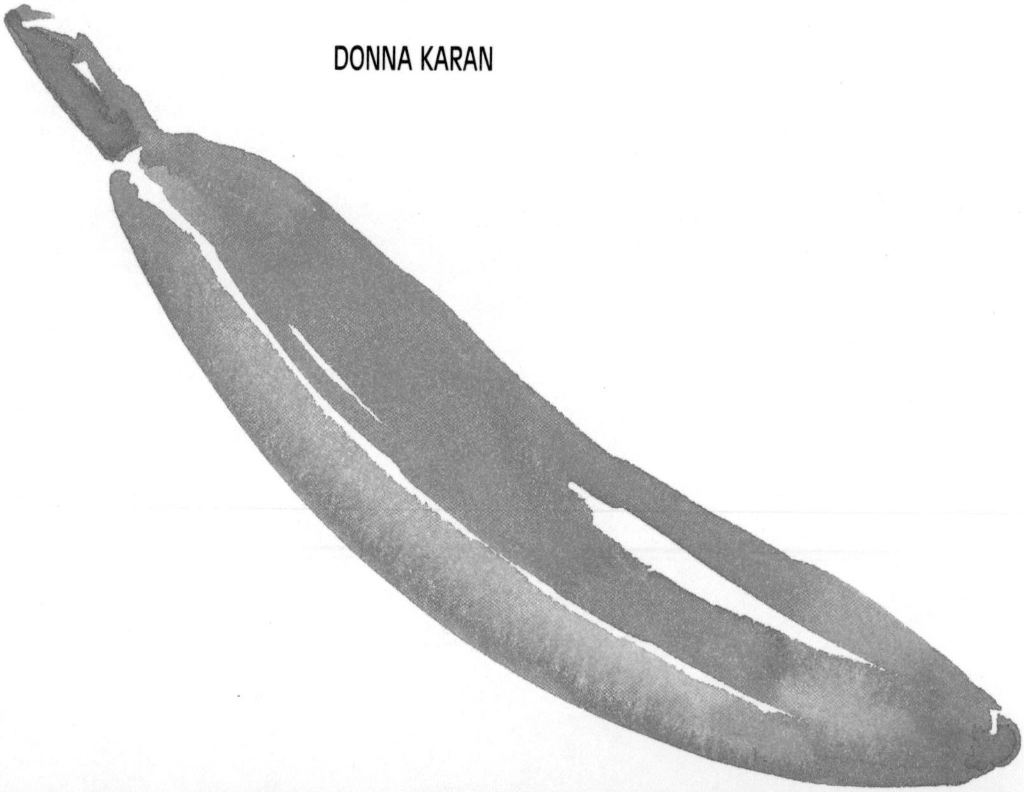

Weight

It's a fact. The books all say here's no way to grow a baby inside, prepare to feed it, and not gain eight. And it also says that when you're born I will lose about thirteen ounds.

I'm eating for two, although you're still no bigger than an elf: It's he idea of you that has a titan's appetite and needs to be fed.

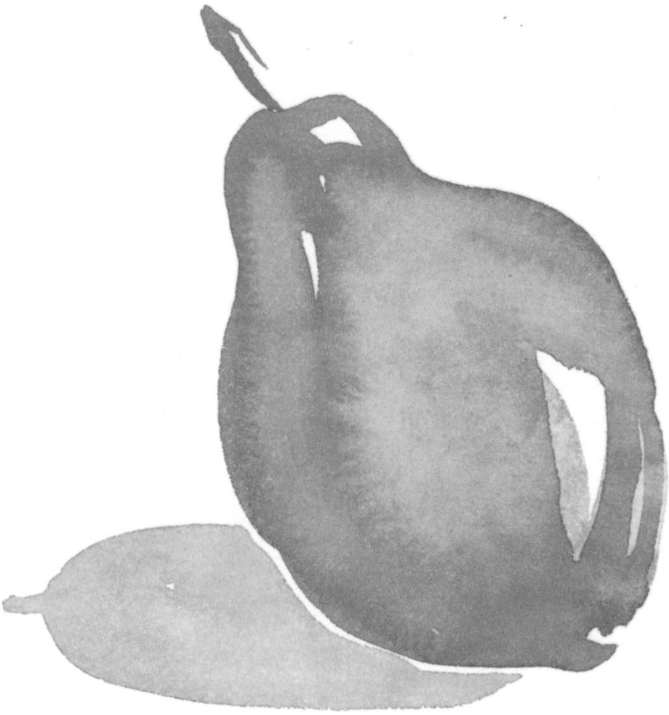

18

18

18

18

What I'd like to wear, my baby, is a hundred-breasted, thousand-jeweled garment of sapphire; a great coat of many colors; disposable gowns flecked with fake precious metals. Large, exotic clothes, to loudly and gorgeously proclaim your passage into being.

Where can I buy such clothes? Where can I wear such clothes?

PHYLLIS CHESLER
With Child, A Diary of Motherhood

Maternity Clothes

Thanks to you, little one, this season brings no pressure to fit into last year's clothes. It is time to improvise styles I've never considered before.

I change clothes as I change roles, and my bold fashion statements will reflect the drama of inner alterations.

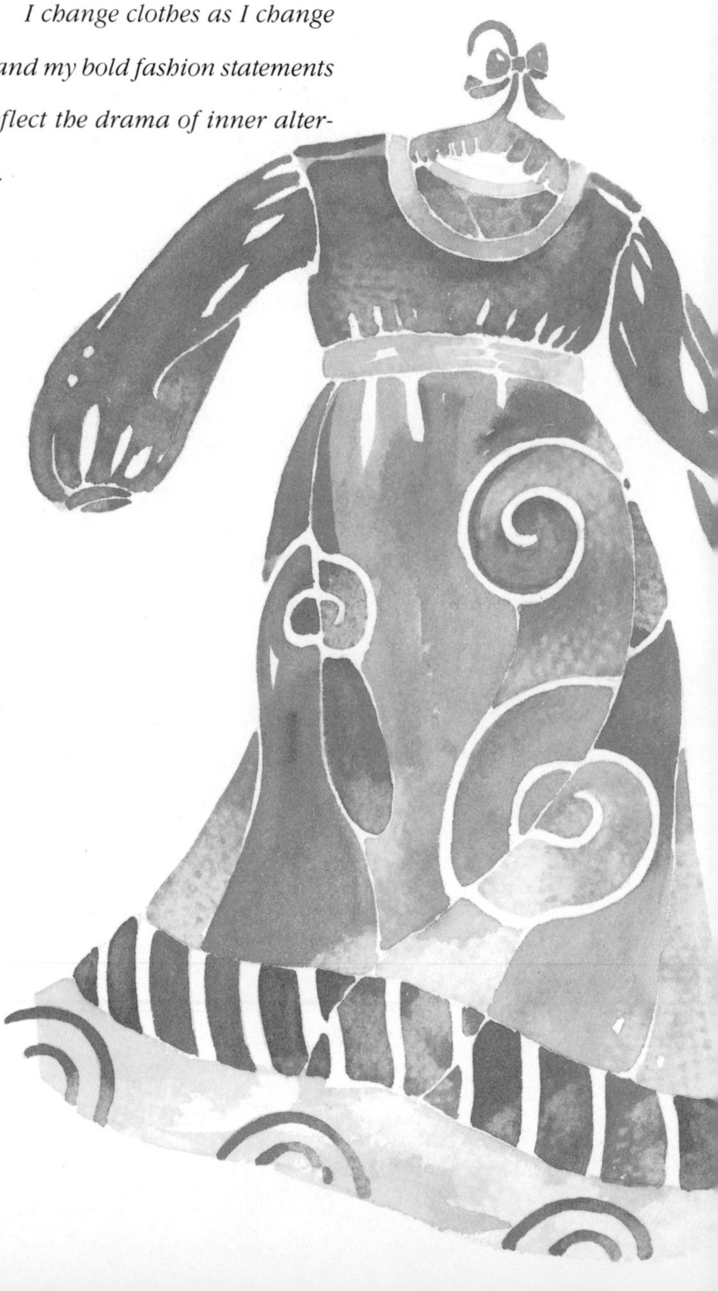

19

19

19

The woman has by now usually put on several pounds, and her abdomen is beginning to be slightly rounded. The upper portion of the uterus has not reached the level of the navel and there is still ample room. Breathing is unaffected, the nausea has ceased and most women find this the best phase of pregnancy, both mentally and physically. A sensation of warmth—as if the body contained a built-in heater—is common.

LENNART NILSSON
A Child Is Born

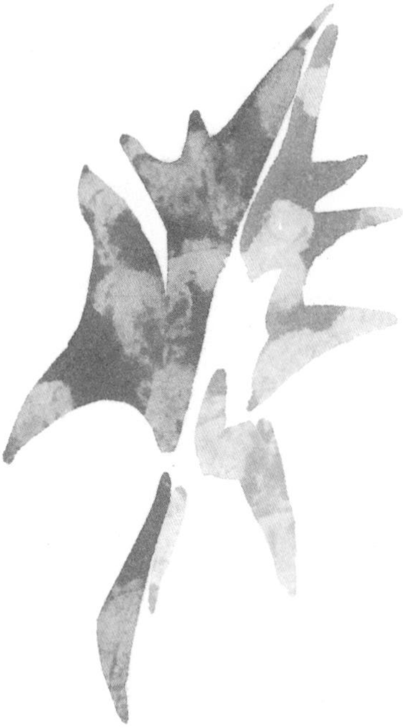

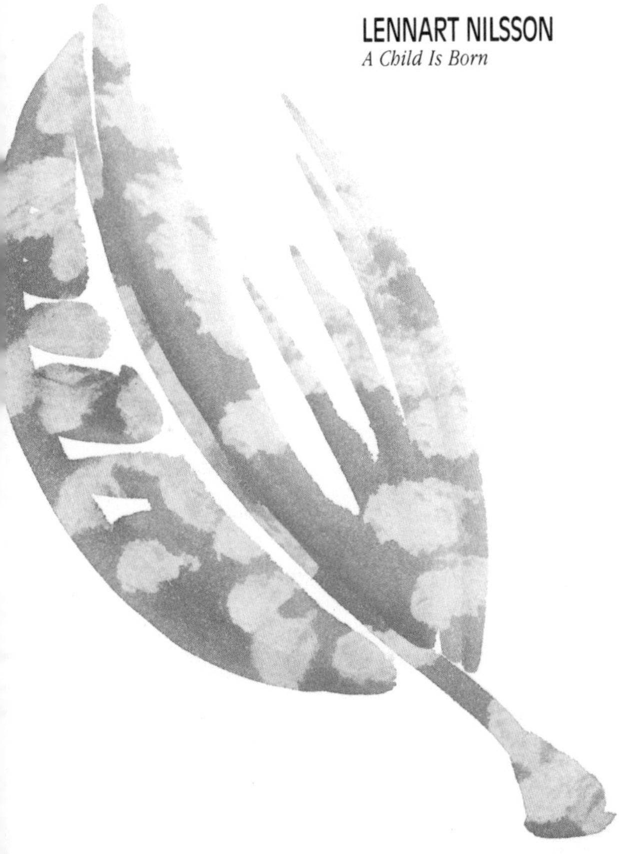

20

Image

I am round-bellied, like th ovum itself, like a picture of the Earth seen from the outer side of its rar atmosphere. I've never looked like this before and didn't know I carrie the potential in me all along.

A pregnant woman is other-worldly, and I suppose that is wh so many people come up and ask to touch my stomach, to make sure I'r still here. They like to give advice, too, I suppose to anchor me on this sia of the gate between the born and the unborn. But, as you know, I hear th whispers of both worlds.

20

20

20

20

Mrs. Darling was married in white, and at first she kept the books perfectly, almost gleefully, as if it were a game, not so much as a Brussels sprout was missing; but by and by whole cauliflowers dropped out, and instead of them there were pictures of babies without faces. She drew them when she should have been totting up. They were Mrs. Darling's guesses.

Wendy came first, then John, then Michael.

JAMES M. BARRIE
Peter Pan

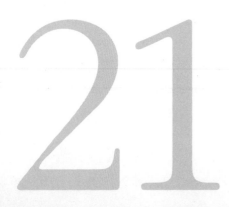

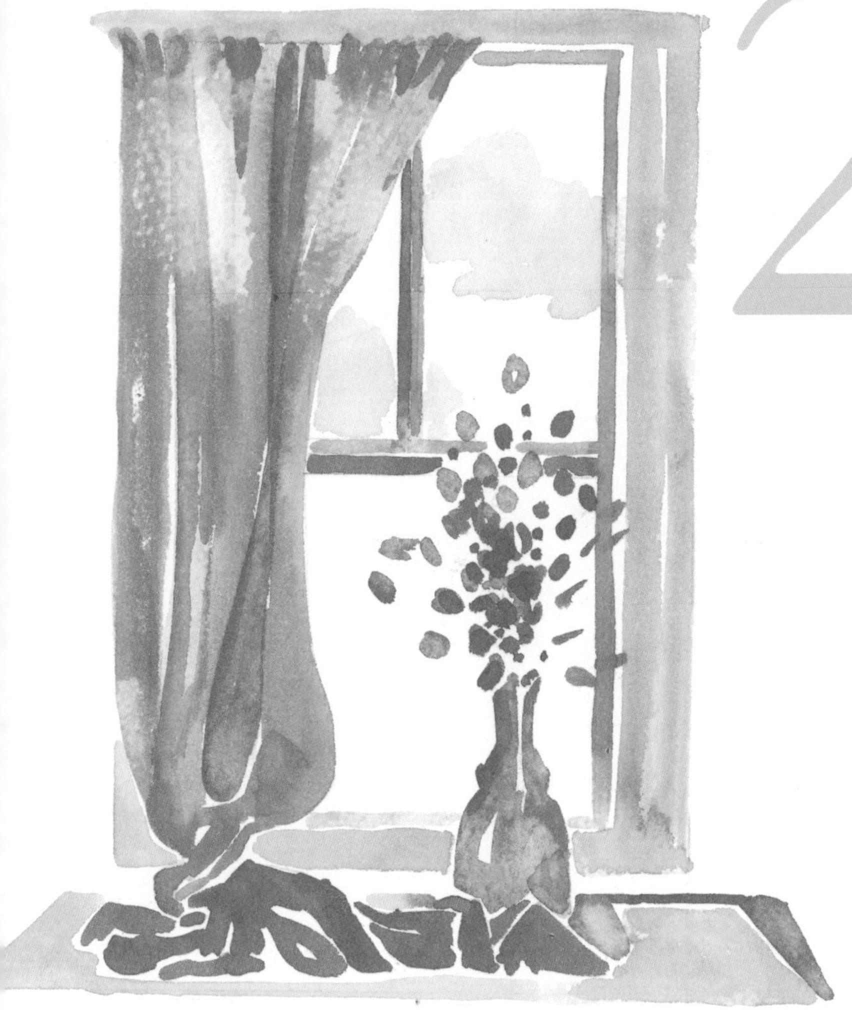

21

D*ear sweet baby, your mother has always been a bit absent-minded, but today I misplaced my wallet and finally found it in the refrigerator.*

It's hard to be in two places at one time.

21

21

21

Movement

22

I have come, Sire, to complain of one of your subjects who has been so audacious as to kick me in the belly.

MARIE ANTOINETTE,
informing her husband, King Louis XVI of France, that she was pregnant with their first child

Movement

22

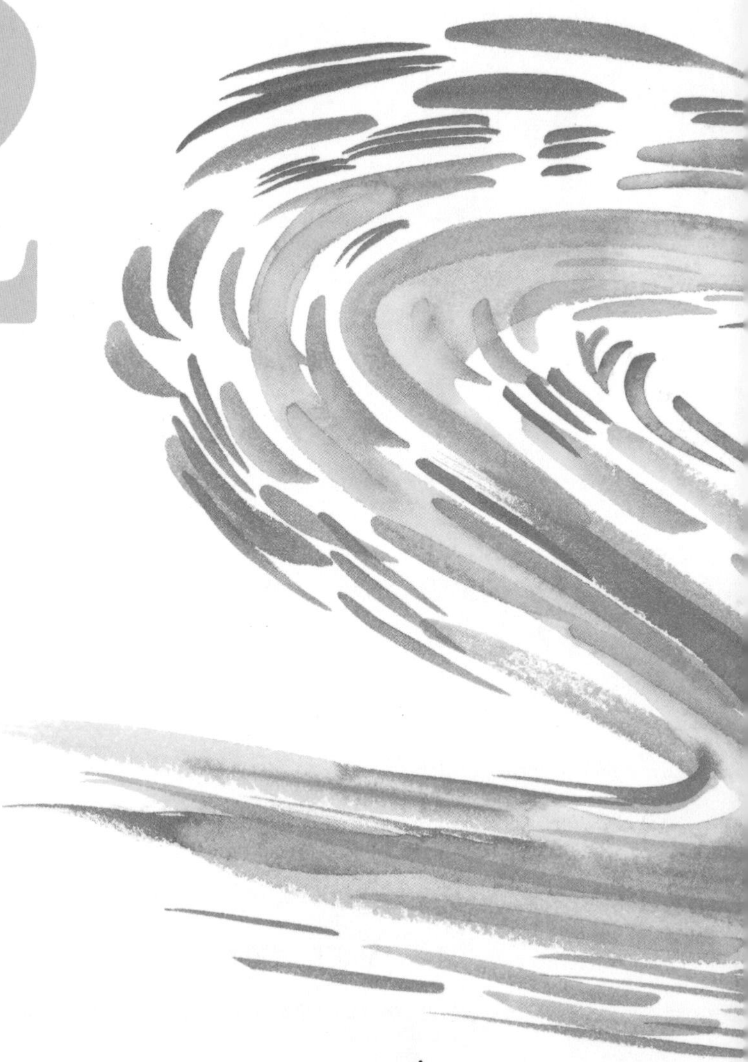

At first it was just a butter

fly's wing that brushed the inside of my stomach. The gentlest flutter, a sigh

But now we celebrate your staccato movements in a wonderfu ritual. It goes like this: Here, here! put your hand here. Now wait, wait feel it? Try there, ahh, feel it?

Take aim, little drummer, now kick!

22

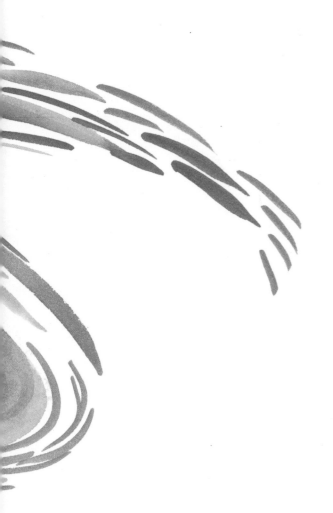

22

22

23

We now know that the unborn child is an aware, reacting human being who from the sixth month on (and perhaps even earlier) leads an active emotional life. Along with this startling finding we have made these discoveries:

The fetus can see, hear, experience, taste and, on a primitive level, even learn in utero (that is, in the uterus—before birth). Most importantly, he can feel—not with an adult's sophistication, but feel nonetheless.

A corollary to this discovery is that what a child feels and perceives begins shaping his attitudes and expectations about himself. . . . The chief source of those shaping messages is the child's mother . . . such life-enhancing emotions as joy, elation and anticipation can contribute significantly to the emotional development of a healthy child. . . .

By and large, the personality of the unborn child a woman bears is a function of the quality of mother-child communication, and also of its specificity. If the communication was abundant, rich, and, most important, nurturing, the chances are very good that the baby will be robust, healthy, and happy.

THOMAS VERNAY, M.D.,
WITH JOHN KELLY
The Secret Life of the Unborn Child

Communication

Intuition suggests—and science now confirms—that the channels of communication open and flow between us, and the placental barrier is no match for the nuances of the mother-infant bond. We are a circle within a circle, and what I give to you spirals back to me as we create each other.

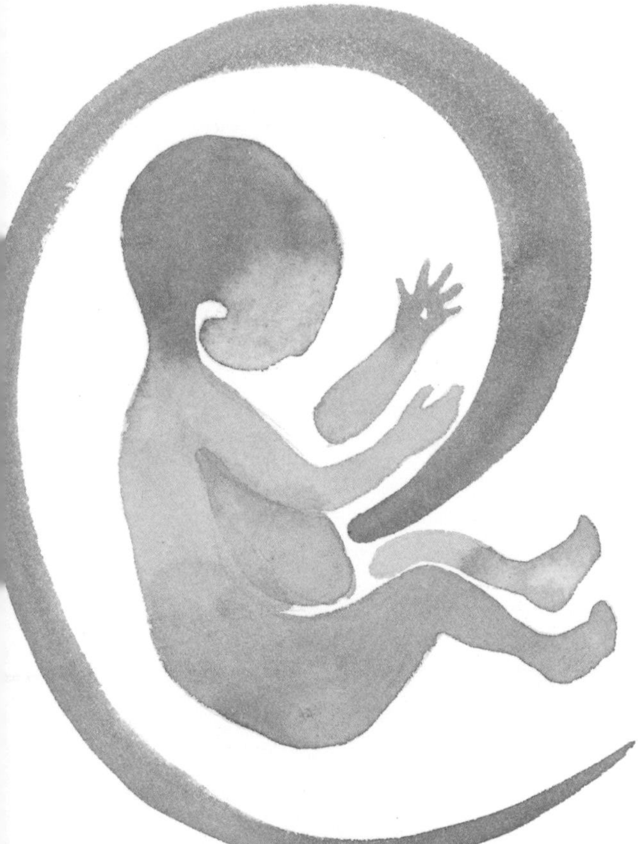

23

23

23

Music

24

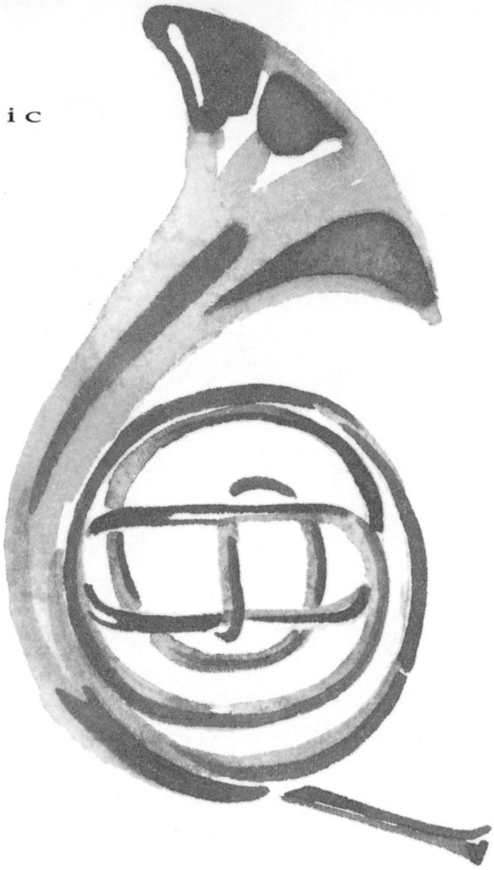

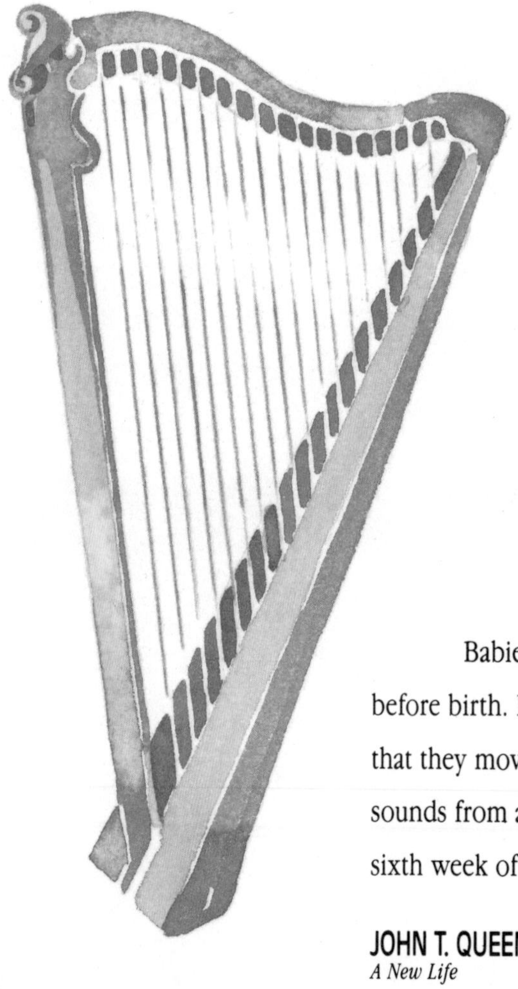

Babies are able to hear long before birth. Research has shown that they move in response to sounds from as early as the twenty-sixth week of pregnancy.

JOHN T. QUEENAN, M.D., ED.
A New Life

Scientists claim that you listen o my heart and the blood pumping through my veins. They say that you ven move your body in rhythm to my speech. I feel you listening to the adio too, and discover that you calm down with Vivaldi, march to Beethoven, and rebel at rock and roll.

And my lullabies? I think we both like the lullabies.

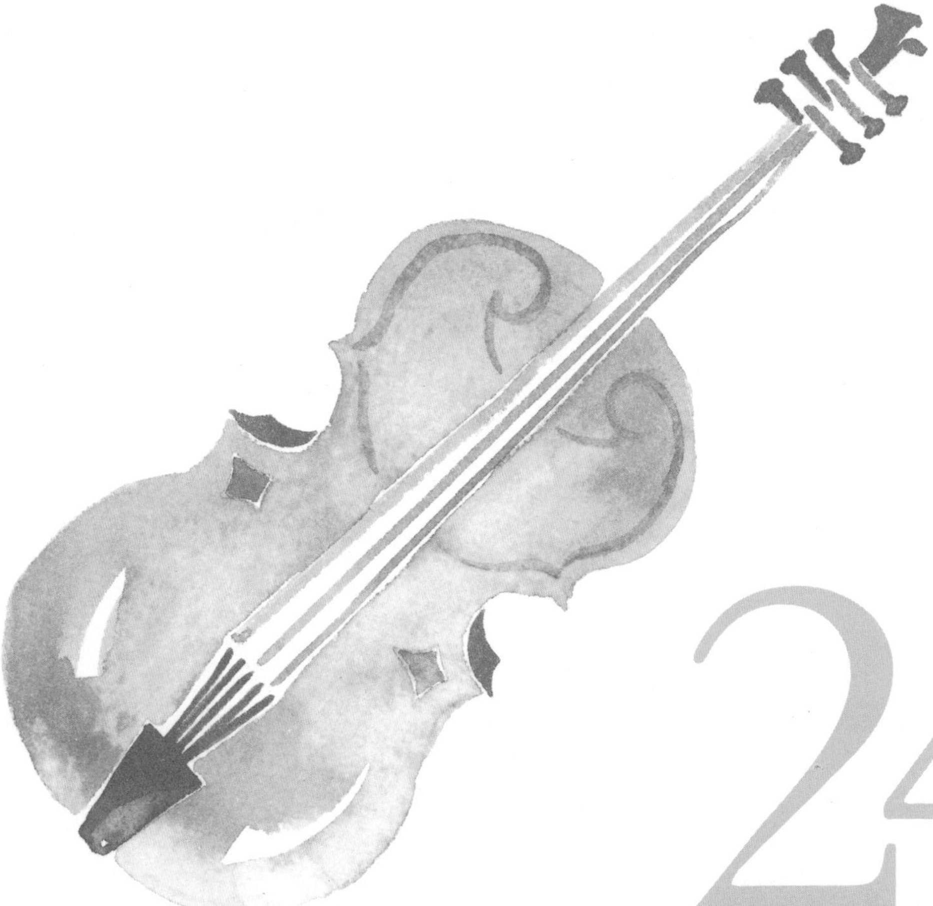

24

24

24

24

The Eyes Open

In the sixth month the eyes can open and the baby can look around.

TRACY HOTCHNER
Pregnancy and Childbirth

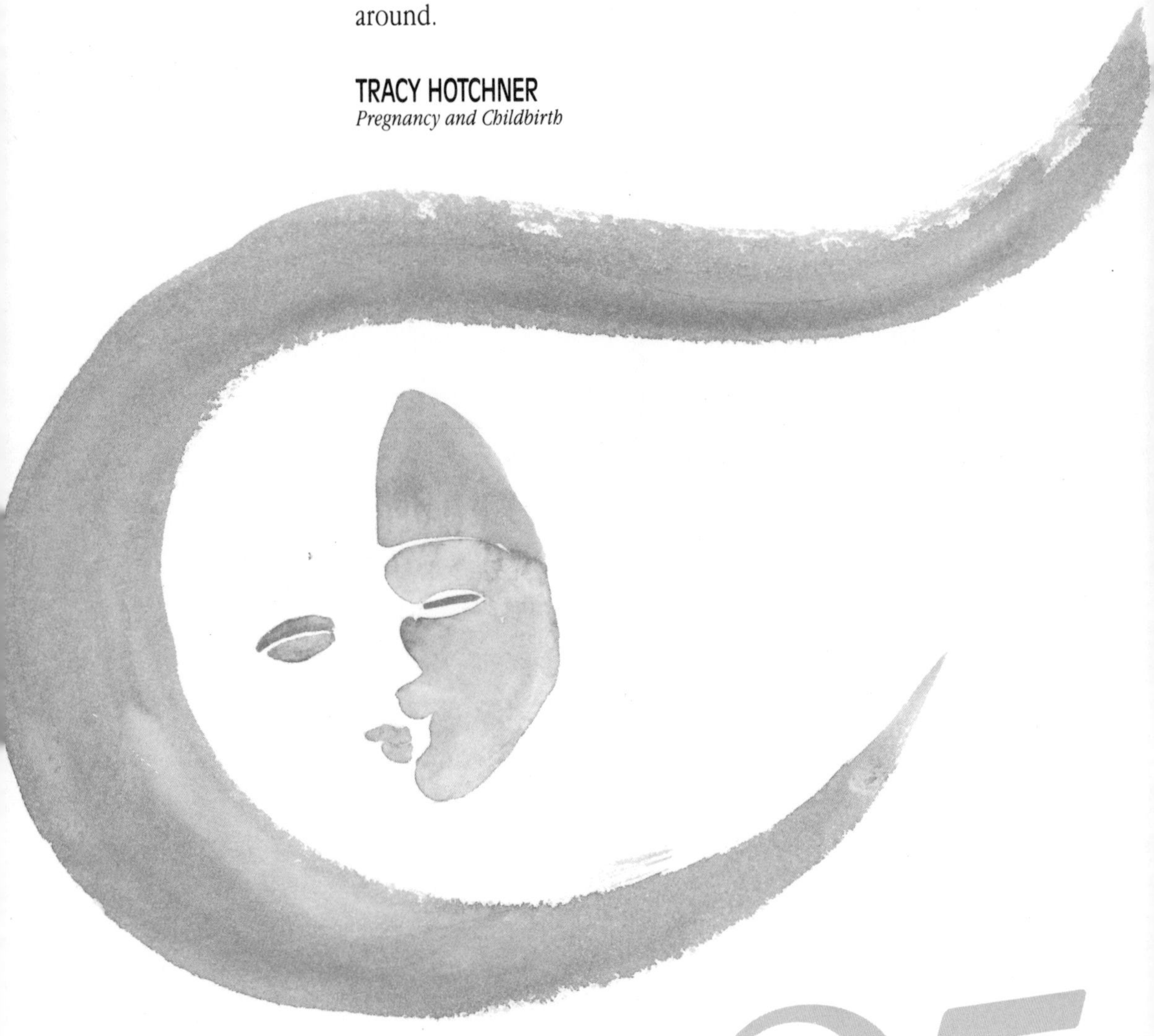

25

If I pass my hand over my stomach, do clouds darken your skies? When you look out at the limits of your world, do starry constellations fleck the dome of my womb?

What do you see? What do you dream?

25

25

25

Insidiously, unhurriedly, the beatitude of pregnant females spread through me. I was no longer subjected to any discomfort, any unease. This purring contentment, this euphoria—how give a name either scientific or familiar to this state of preservation?—must certainly have penetrated me, since I have not forgotten it and am recalling it now, when life can never again bring me plenitude.

Every night I bade farewell, more or less, to one of the happiest periods of my life, knowing well how I was going to regret it. But the cheerfulness, the purring contentment, the euphoria submerged everything and over me reigned the sweet animal innocence and unconcern arising from my added weight and the muffled appeals of the new life being formed within me.

COLETTE
Earthly Paradise

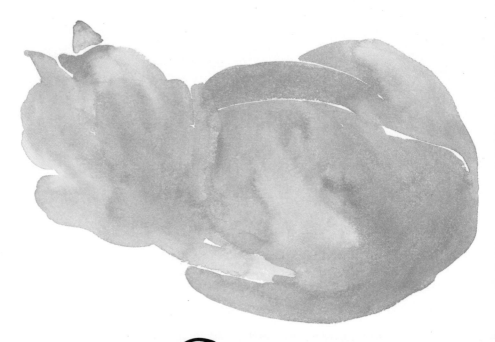

Colette wrote this at the age of forty, when she was pregnant with her first and only child. I understand that wonderful phrase, "purring contentment."

Each pregnancy is so different, and so similar.

26

26

26

26

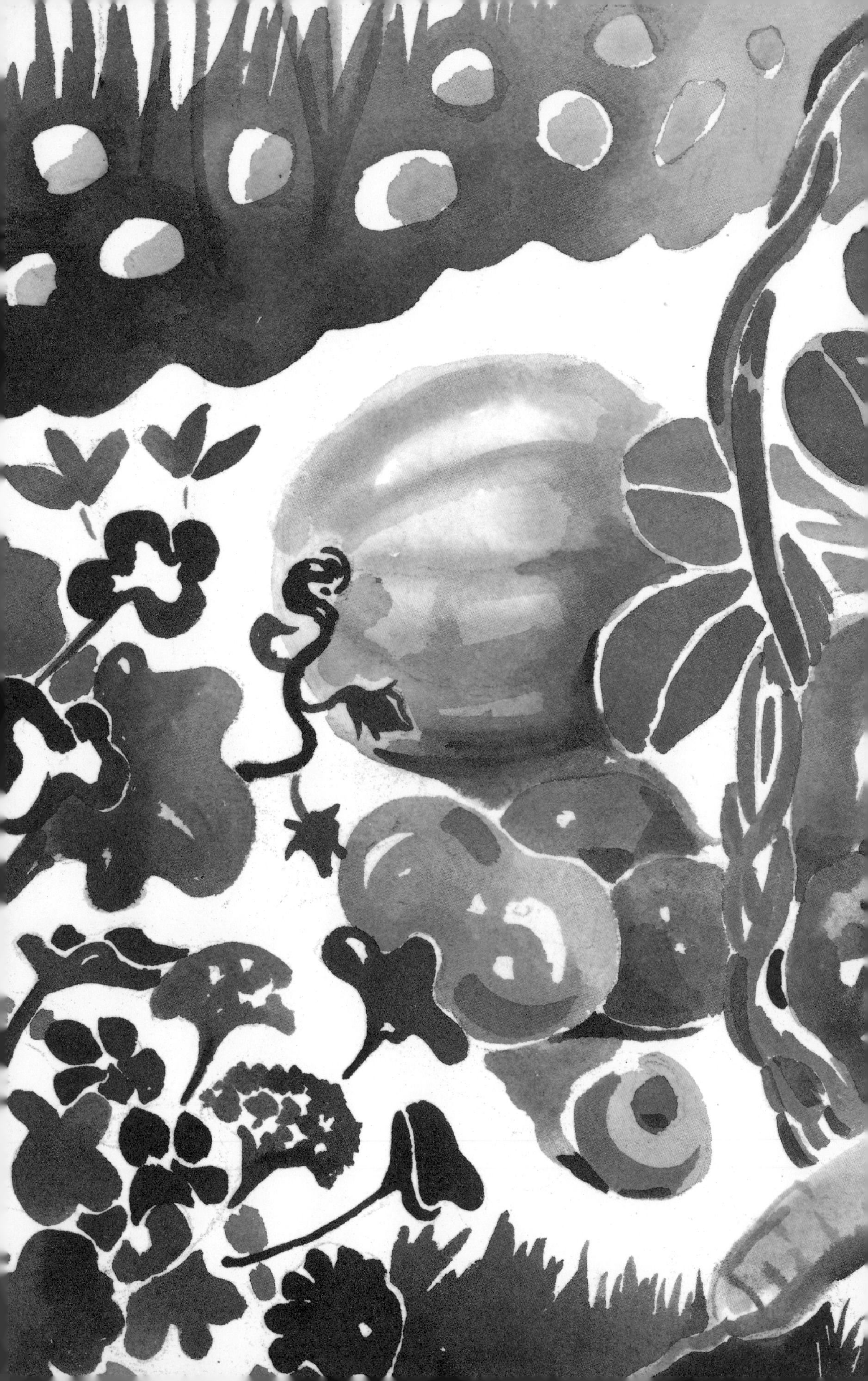

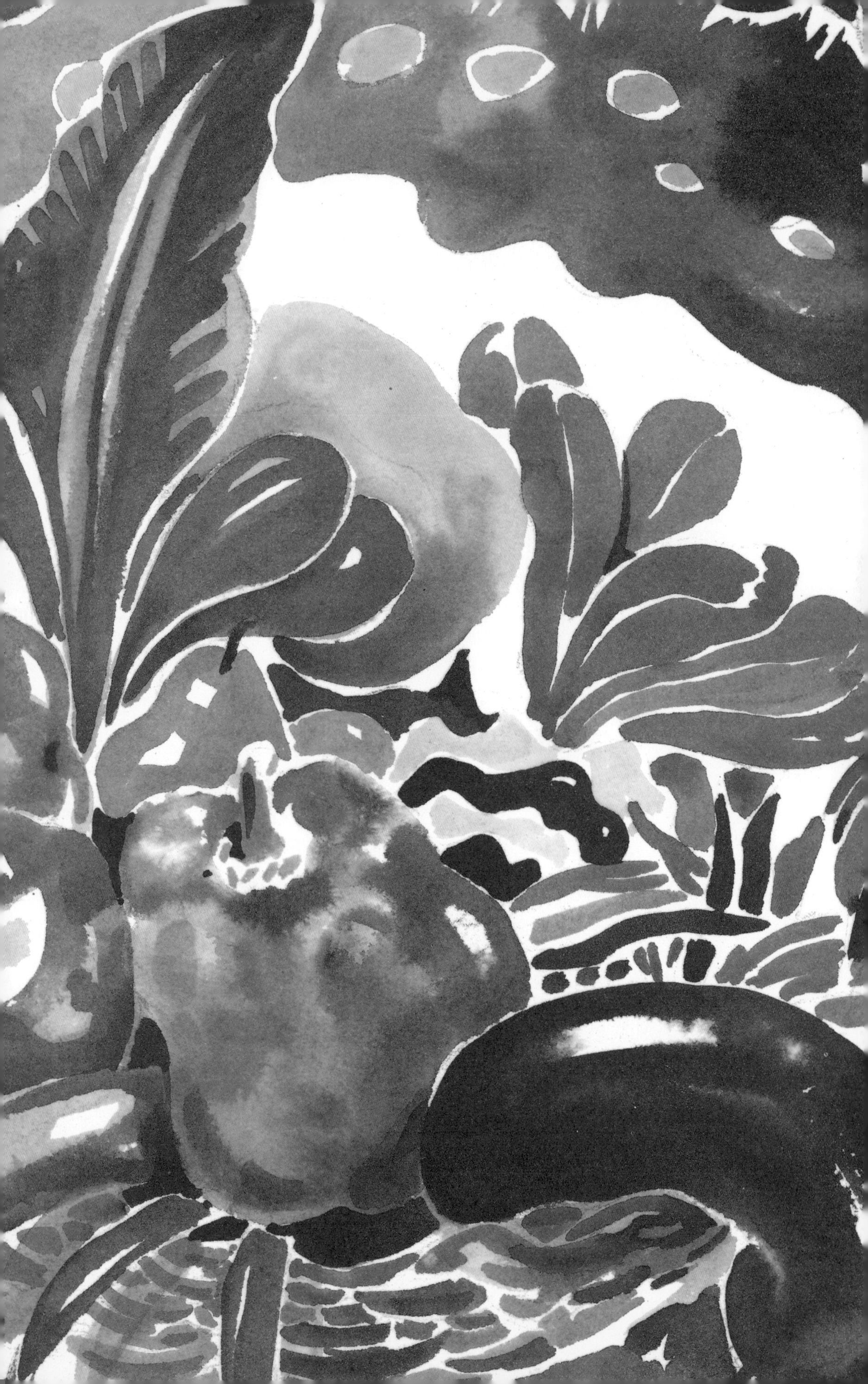

Visibility

During pregnancy, a man is sort of oblivious to how it has taken over a woman's life. Your colleagues at the office are aware that you are expecting a child; but they don't let it get in the way of the work routine.

Today, though, Susan asked me to go to the grocery store where she usually shops to pick up some sandwiches for lunch. I did; as soon as I walked in, the man behind the meat counter said, "I take i this means she had her baby."

Some other women who were shopping said, "Susan had her baby?" Bud, the owner, called from behind the cash register: "Boy or girl?"

When I told him, the butcher overheard and said, "I lost my bet."

In the nine months of her pregnancy, I had never been in here it had never occurred to me that the news meant anything to anyone outside our own home. But of course, everywhere a pregnant woman goes she is advertising the coming event.

BOB GREENE
Good Morning, Merry Sunshine

27

Visibility

27

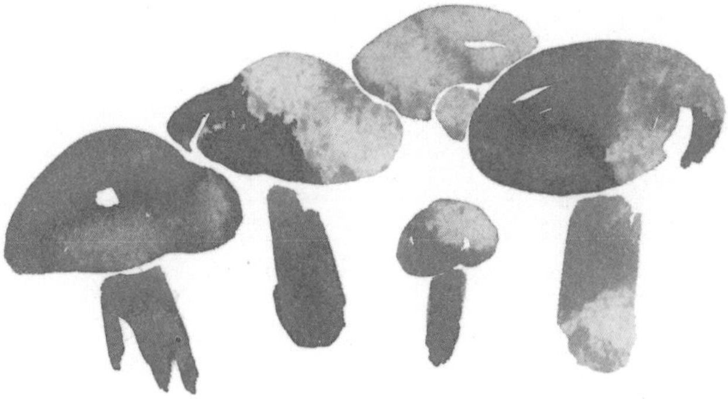

Is it true that men do not see pregnant women? I see them everywhere. They were never there before—well, maybe one or two, but not the swollen-ankled, tent-draped armies I see now. Perhaps there's been a population explosion, or perhaps because of cabin fever we've all taken to the streets in collective bursts.

27

27

The first cradle was within the mother, and children in their metaphorical genius relive the experience over and over through play and rhyme—falling on the hard ground together. "Down will come baby, cradle and all," is an externalization of the process of being born, of coming down to earth.

LAURA CHESTER
Cradle and All

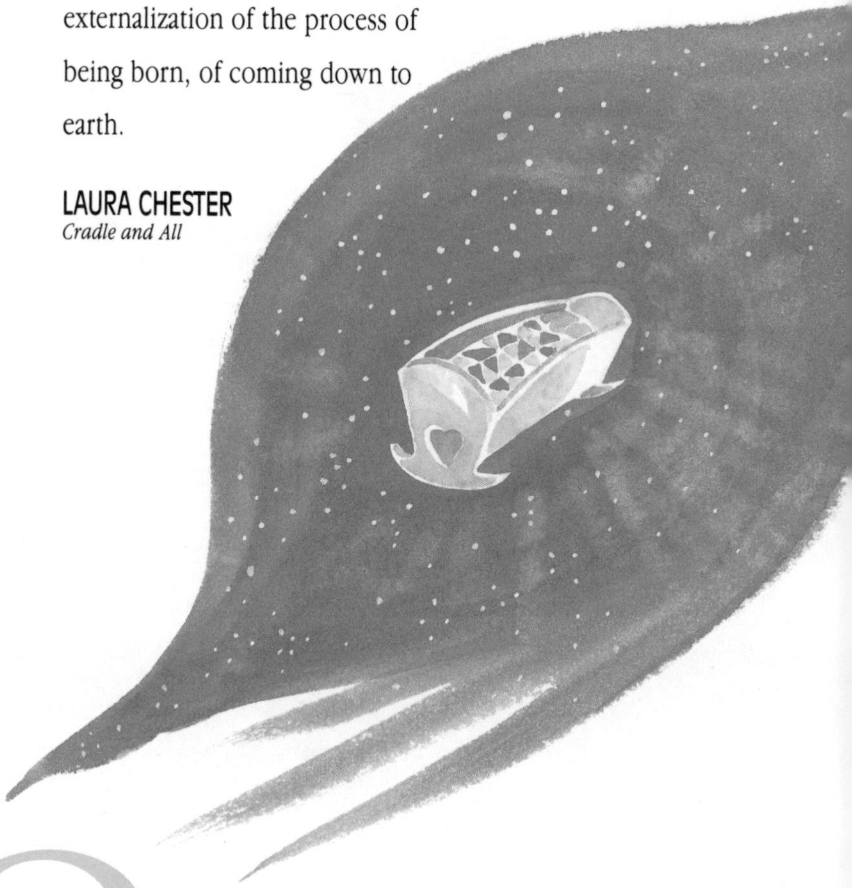

28

Viability

28

Twenty-eight weeks brings a celebration. If you were born at this point, you could live on your own. Your first step toward independence and separation. Now you look to me not for creation but nurturance. And I keep you close as long as you need it, to stuff you fat with love, to make the world a softer place.

My cradle rocks you still, and after the bough breaks, another milestone of independence, I will catch you in my arms.

28

28

28

29

She would have no one with her when the hour came. It came one night, early, when the sun was scarcely set. She was working beside him in the harvest field. The wheat had borne and been cut and the field flooded and the young rice set, and now the rice bore harvest, and the ears were ripe and full after the summer rains and the warm ripening sun of early autumn. Together they cut the sheaves all day, bending and cutting with short-handled scythes. She had stooped stiffly, because of the burden she bore, and she moved more slowly than he, so that they cut unevenly, his row ahead, and hers behind. . . . She stopped and stood up then, her scythe dropped. On her face was a new sweat, the sweat of a new agony.

"It is come," she said. "I will go into the house. Do not come into the room until I call. Only bring me a newly peeled reed, and slit it, that I may cut the child's life from mine."

PEARL S. BUCK
The Good Earth

29

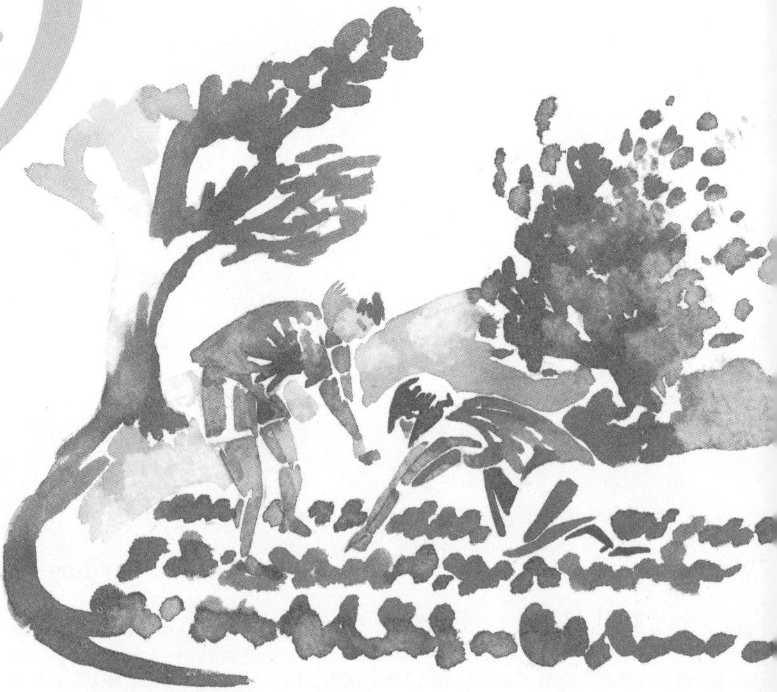

We have decisions to make: home, hospital, or rice paddy—definitely not rice paddy! Lamaze or Grantly Dick-Reade, Bradley or epidural.

Did you know that Jimmy Carter was the first United States President to be born in a hospital, and the rest, from George Washington right up to Gerald Ford, were born at home?

29

29

30

On January 19, 1847, Scottish physician James Young Simpson plashed a half teaspoonful of chloroform on a handkerchief and held it ver the nose of a laboring woman.

Less than half an hour later, she became the first woman to eliver while under anesthesia. (There was only one complication: Vhen the woman—whose first baby had been born after three days of ainful labor—awoke, Dr. Simpson was unable to convince her that he'd actually given birth.)

RLENE EISENBERG, HEIDI EISENBERG IURKOFF, AND SANDEE EISENBERG IATHAWAY, R.N., B.S.N.
'hat to Expect When You're Expecting

Anesthesia

30

Birth is not an Olympic event, and no one is giving out medals for the best performance. There is only one goal for us in all of this—to make it safely through. And whether you come after three hours of labor or spring full-grown from my forehead like Pallas Athena, it does not matter to me.

30

30

30

31

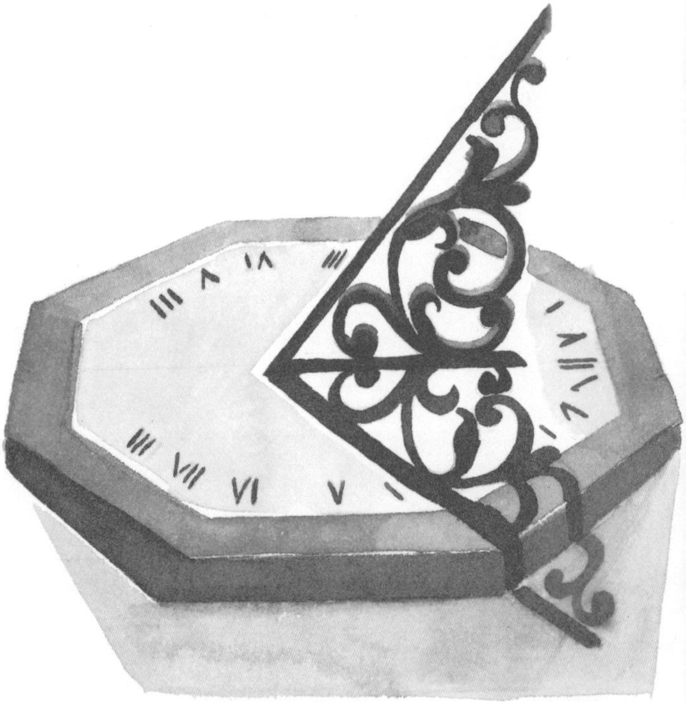

We are shown a final movie about birth. As each baby emerges from the mother, the sound track plays a burst of religious organ music. I cry on cue at each delivery. There is now such a strong link in me between deliveries and tears, I believe I would cry at the receipt of a special delivery letter.

DAN GREENBURG
Confessions of a Pregnant Father

So much of my reading now s about pregnancy and birth—preparation (the trips to the doctor), suspense (and then the mother woke up with a twinge), drama (the white-nuckled breathing of labor, heart monitors), and then, her deliverance. know the plot by heart, and yet I read on and on, fact and fiction, and each time, just at the climax ("it's a——baby!"), I am full up.

It comes from somewhere just above where you rest, wells up through the throat, tightens the jaw, and is released in a wash of tears. And cry, the tears blocking my vision, and I have to wait in the vicarious blind emotion of the moment until I can read again (and they put the baby on her stomach and she held her child in her arms for the first time).

31

31

31

32

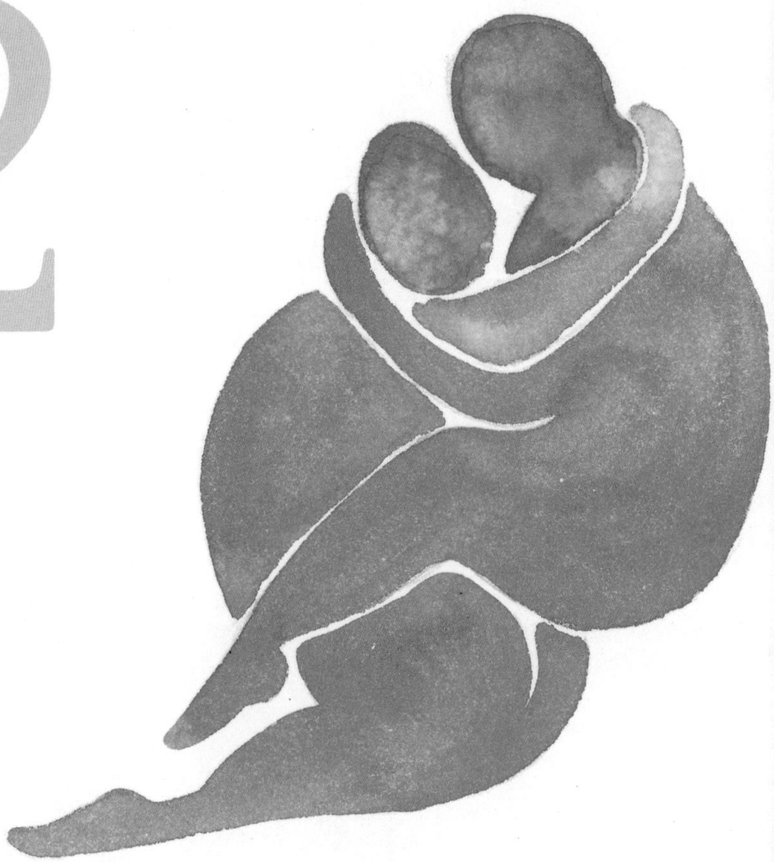

No one ever told you there would be such tedium and listlessness, such queer aches and fancies. You were prepared for the queasiness, which is common, and the craving for odd food, like pickles, which is not, but no one ever told you how much you would want to make love, and how silly you would look when you did.

MARGUERITE KELLY AND ELIA PARSONS
The Mother's Almanac

This is a fill-in-the-blank. Making love after you're pregnant is like ____________________?

Your father said, "like scrambling eggs without breaking the shell." I think that means he wants to be very, very gentle with both of us.

I think it's like the moon and stars on a fine night. One has basically nothing to do with the other, except to enhance the sky.

32

32

32

That is why I had children: to offer them a perfect dream of childhood that can fill their soul as they grow older. . .

ANNA QUINDLEN
Living Out Loud

A baby is God's opinion that life should go on.

CARL SANDBURG

. . . And yet I love this little life! With all the pain of it, I long for the wonderful thing to happen, for a tiny human creature to spring from between my limbs bravely out into the world, I need it, just as a true poet needs to create a great undying work.

YANG PING
"Fragment from a Lost Diary"

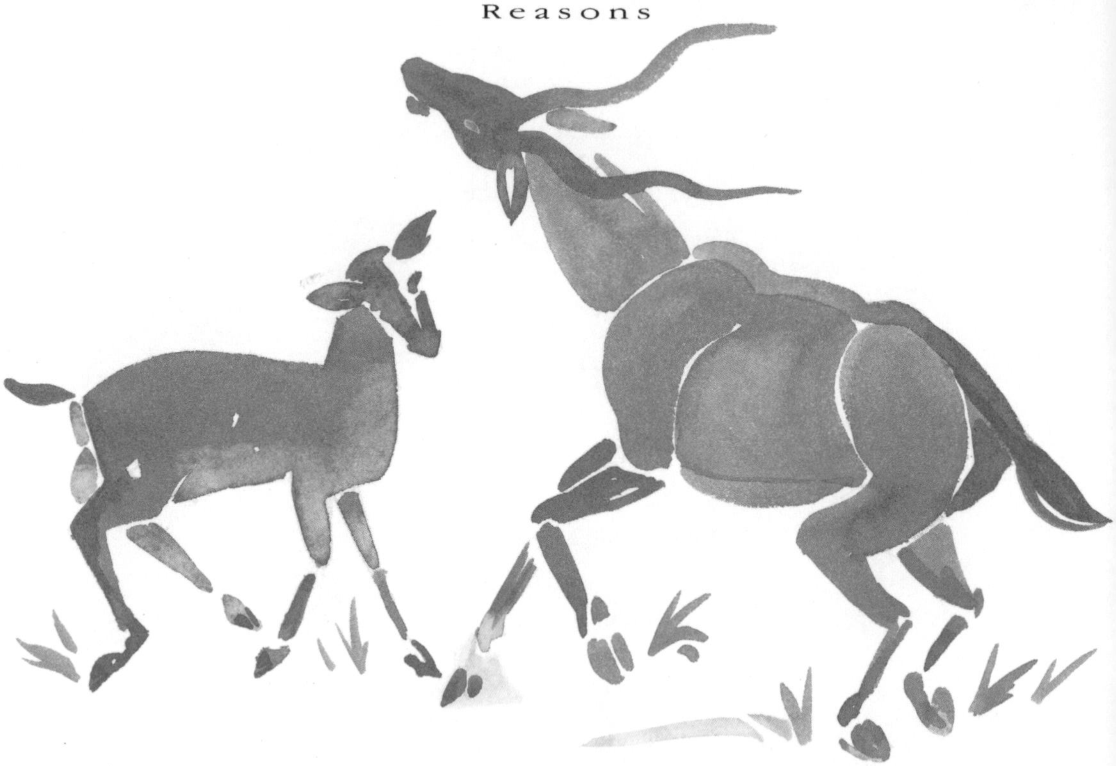

I take my body with me on because I can't leave it behind. I can't see my feet, and I am a collectio of odd sensations.

I wrap my arms around my huge stomach in order to cradle yo and I know the decision to give birth has absolutely nothing to do wit reason.

33

33

33

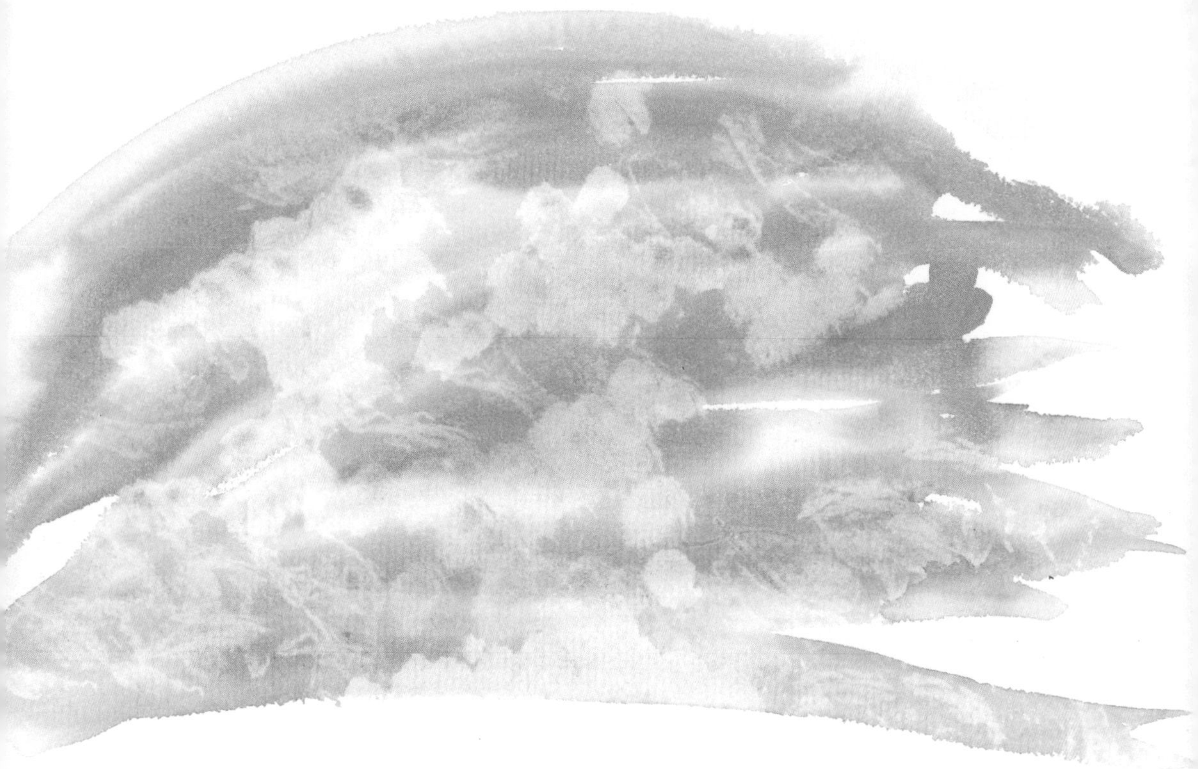

How I tumbled into dreams after that, hugging the fatly anonymous hospital pillow, dreaming the lips of babies, that sucking pull, the sigh and swallow, dreaming the nights ahead when each fine-tuned whimper would pull me back to earth, unfolding fists around a finger, dreaming the earth's secret rattle as it turned in space on its ancient implacable hinge.

NAOMI SHIHAB NYE
"The Rattle of Wheels Toward the Rooms of the New Mothers"

34

Heavy with child, my mind trips through nightly gymnastics.

Sometimes frightening, always fantastic; I discover a sea of dreams in my pouch.

34

34

34

Margaret Mead paid me a visit today . . . she insisted on coming to see me, because "being pregnant is more fragile a state than being old." As she comes in, . . . her first question, before we sit down is: "What are you doing about your nipples?". . . I say: "Nothing."

"Rub them with a rough washcloth, pinch them, toughen them up," she tells me. Bluntly. Simply.

PHYLLIS CHESLER
With Child, A Diary of Motherhood

35

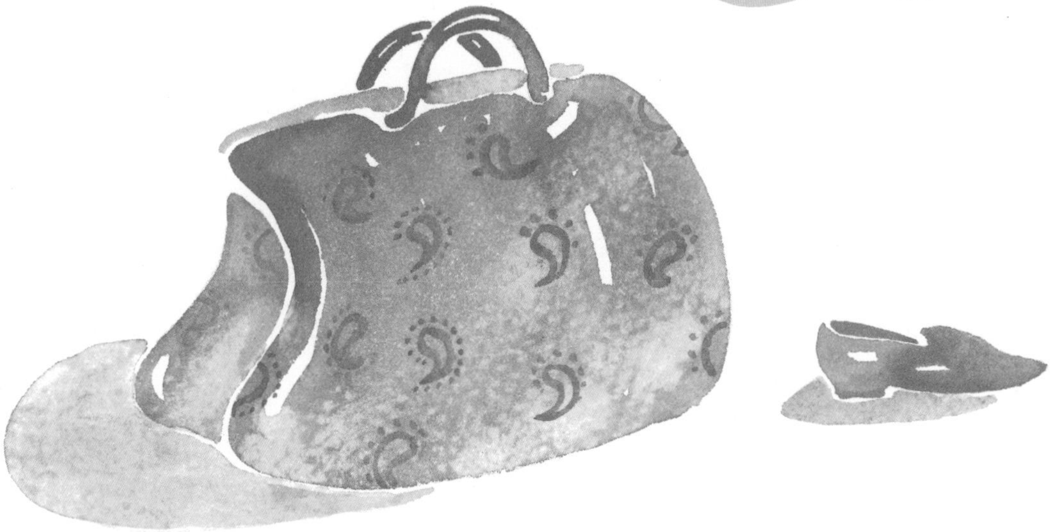

I *prepare for a great trip and gather bits and pieces and put them in a sack.*

"This is what you'll need," the books say, and list a drug store assortment of silly items: lollipops and perfume, stamps and a camera.

In fact, we need nothing at all except that which we are. We are like a child's Christmas present—all parts included, and now, assembly complete.

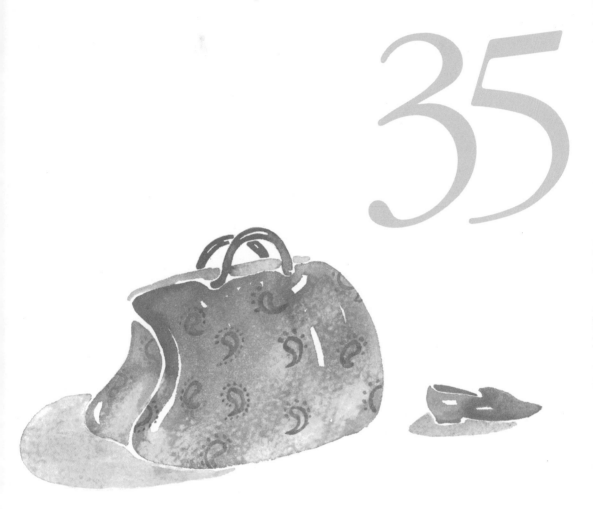

35

35

If pregnancy were a book they would cut the last two chapters.

NORA EPHRON

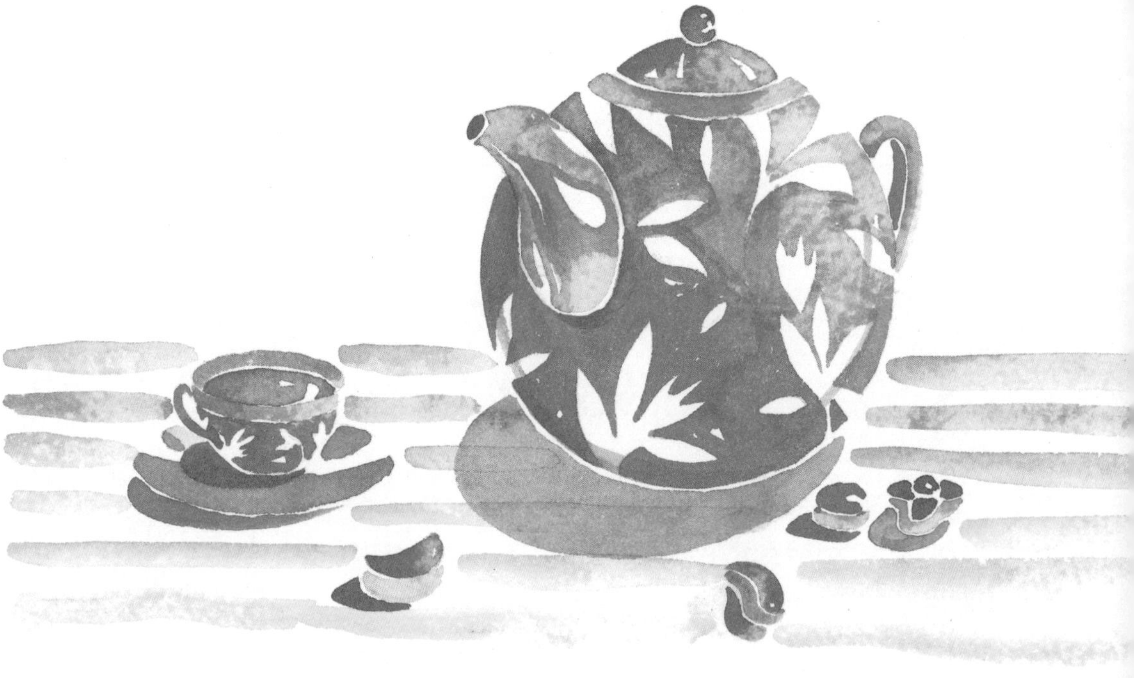

36

I can practically see your knees and count your toes. I feel that this pregnancy has been as long as recorded history.

Actually, I don't know why I'm in such a hurry. A friend of a friend looked at my stomach and said, "Don't rush; it's the best babysitter you'll ever have."

36

36

36

37

The strange part is what follows. That as the full-term pregnant woman sits, face to the sun, in a calm tidal pool, staring out to a sea with not a whitecap in sight, suddenly—she never knows when—there comes a tidal wave. I have known plenty of women to dread the birth, and afterward to curse the agony they went through. For myself, I look forward to the event with the anticipation of a passionate surfer. More accurately, with the anticipation of one who never could surf, or ski, or stay on a skateboard even. The last one chosen for every school field hockey and basketball team she ever played on. Before I had children I always wondered whether their births would be, for me, like the ultimate in my gym class failures. And discovered, instead (no particular skill evident here, except maybe concentration), that I'd finally found my sport. . . .

I love riding the wave of childbirth—love even how hard it is, and when the moment comes that I know I've done it for the last time, I'll mourn. But giving birth is an experience and parenthood is a state of being; the one passes, the other never ends.

JOYCE MAYNARD
Hers, Through Women's Eyes

37

Parenthood is quite a long word. I expect it contains the rest of my life.

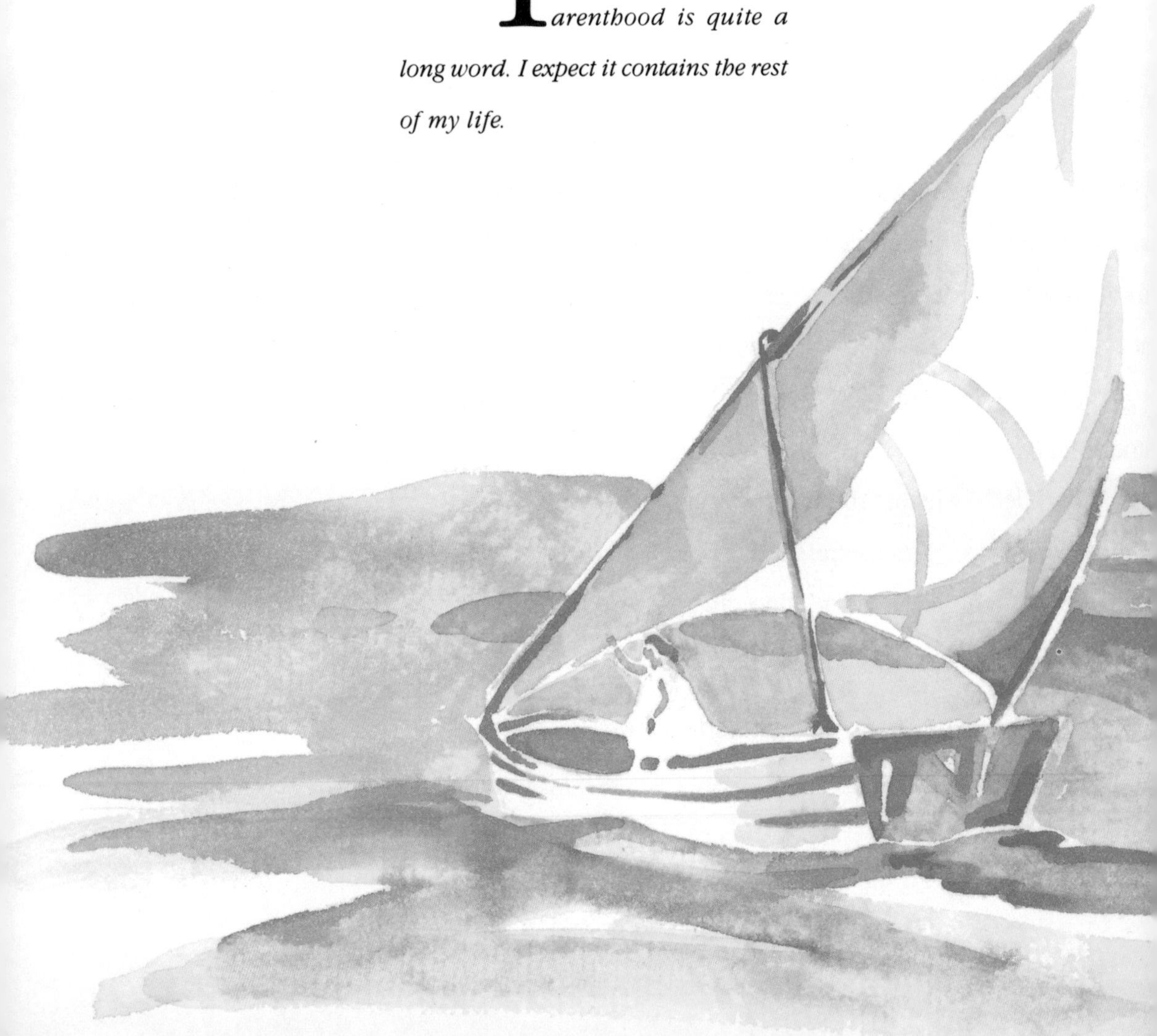

37

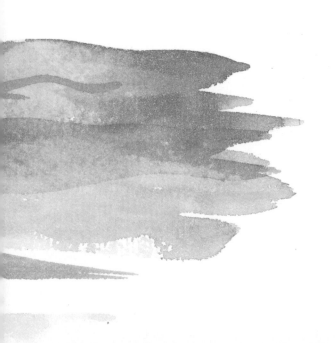

37

38

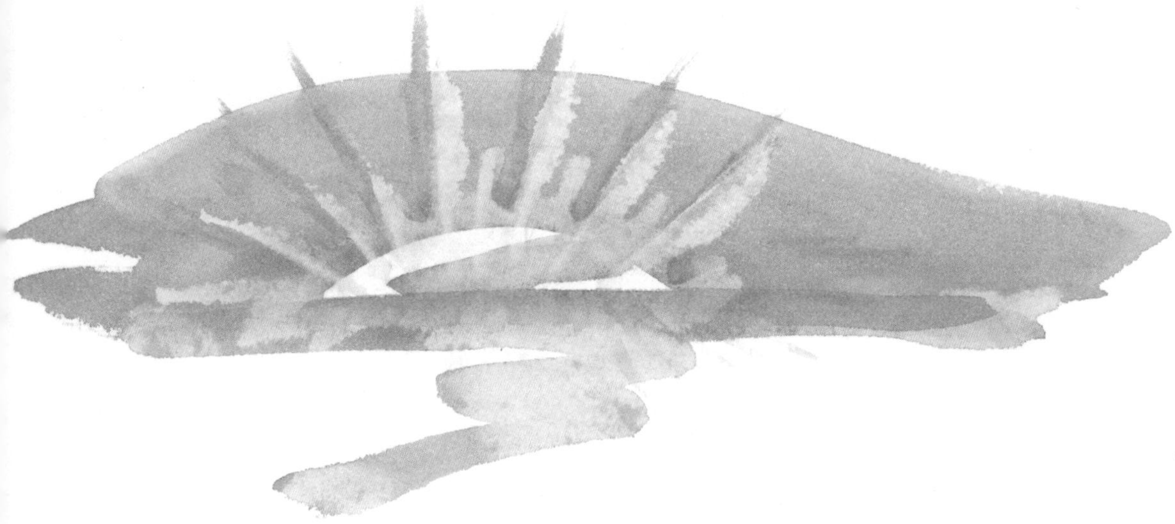

The instant of birth is exquisite.
Pain and joy are one at this moment.
Ever after, the dim recollection is
so sweet that we speak to our children
with a gratitude they never understand.

MADELINE TIGER
"Birth"

A Birth

38

Women trade birth experiences as men trade war stories. These women warriors go to battle to create life and that, I think, is a war we win.

38

38

38

39

as I had
ridden down toward the light with my lips
pressed against the sides of that valve in her body,
she was
bearing down and then breathing in the mask and then
bearing down, pressing me out into the
world that was not enough for her without me in it,
not the moon, the sun, the stars, Orion,
cartwheeling easily across the dark, not the
earth, the sea, none of it was
enough for her, without me.

SHARON OLDS
"The Planned Child"

why wasn't the room bursting with lilies? why was
everything the same with them moving so slowly as if
they were drugged? why were they acting the same
when
suddenly, everything had changed?

TOI DERRICOTTE
"Natural Birth"

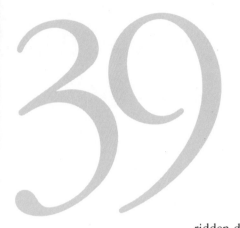

A Baby

Suddenly, there is one more person in the room, and you didn't come in through the door. I realize we've known each other for a long long time, and my little swimmer is now dancing.

As I nurse you, I am humbled, speechless, and my body sings.

Thank you.

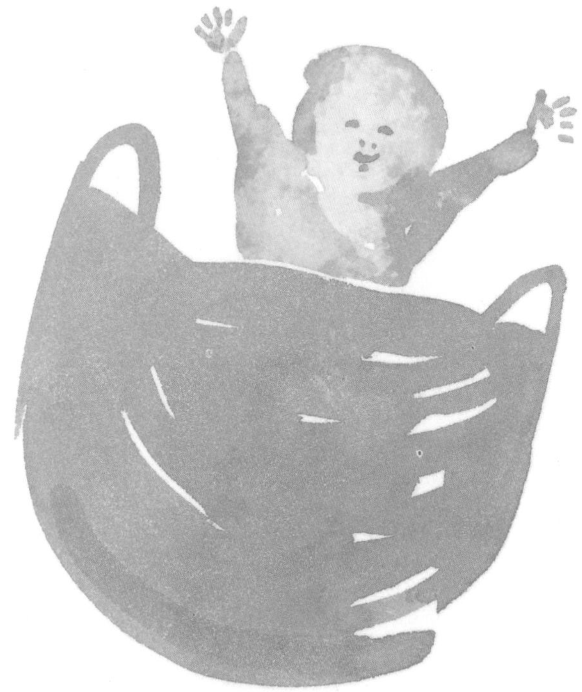

39

39

39

40

I have done what you wanted to do, Walt
Whitman,
Allen Ginsberg, I have done this thing,
I and the other women this exceptional
act with the exceptional heroic body,
this giving birth, this glistening verb,
and I am putting my proud American boast
right here with the others.

SHARON OLDS
"The Language of the Brag"

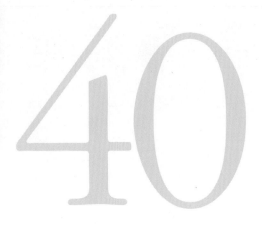

A Brag

40

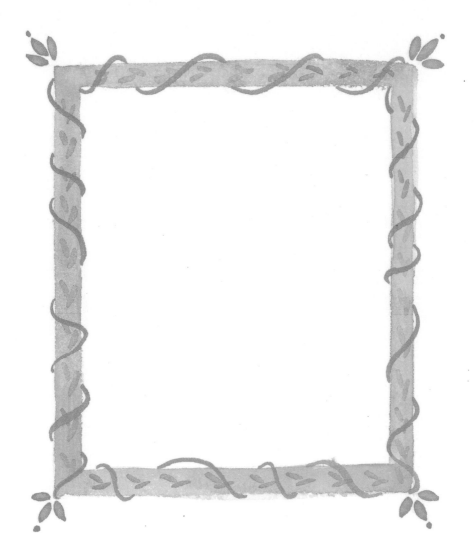

40

40